Obstetrics and Gynecology

Notice

Medicine is an ever-changing science. As new research and clinical experience broaden our knowledge, changes in treatment and drug therapy are required. The editors and the publisher of this work have made every effort to ensure that the drug dosage schedules herein are accurate and in accord with the standards accepted at the time of publication. Readers are advised, however, to check the product information sheet included in the package of each drug they plan to administer to be certain that changes have not been made in the recommended dose or in the contraindications for administration. This recommendation is of particular importance in connection with new or infrequently used drugs.

Obstetrics and Gynecology:

PreTest® Self-Assessment and Review

Third Edition

Editor

Mark I. Evans, M.D.
Director, Division of Reproductive Genetics
Assistant Professor of Obstetrics
and Gynecology
Wayne State University
Hutzel Hospital
Detroit, Michigan

McGraw-Hill Book Company
Health Professions Division
PreTest Series

New York   St. Louis   San Francisco
Auckland   Bogotá   Guatemala   Hamburg
Johannesburg   Lisbon   London   Madrid
Mexico   Montreal   New Delhi   Panama
Paris   San Juan   São Paulo   Singapore
Sydney   Tokyo   Toronto

Library of Congress Cataloging in Publication Data
Main entry under title:

Obstetrics and gynecology: PreTest self-assessment and
    review.

    Second ed. edited by William H. Swartz.
    Bibliography: p.
    1. Gynecology—Examinations, questions, etc.
2. Obstetrics—Examinations, questions, etc. 1. Evans,
Mark I. [DNLM: 1. Gynecology—examination questions.
2. Obstetrics—examination questions. WP 18 014]
RG111.037   1985   618'.076   84-12572
ISBN 0-07-051001-6

34567890   HULHUL   898765

ISBN 0-07-051001-6

This book was set in English Times (Times Roman) by Allen Wayne Communica-
tions, Inc.; the editors were Beth Ann Kaufman and Irene Curran; the production
supervisor was Avé McCracken.
The Hull Printing Co., Inc. was printer and binder.

Contents

Introduction

Obstetrics and Gynecology: PreTest Self-Assessment and Review, 3rd Ed., has been designed to provide medical students, as well as physicians, with a comprehensive and convenient instrument for self-assessment and review within the field of obstetrics and gynecology. The 500 questions provided have been designed to parallel the format and degree of difficulty of the questions contained in Part II of the National Board of Medical Examiners examinations, the Federation Licensing Examination (FLEX), and the Foreign Medical Graduate Examination in the Medical Sciences (FMGEMS).

Each question in the book is accompanied by an answer, a paragraph explanation, and a specific page reference to either a current journal article, a textbook, or both. A bibliography that lists all the sources used in the book follows the last chapter.

Perhaps the most effective way to use this book is to allow yourself one minute to answer each question in a given chapter; as you proceed, indicate your answer beside each question. By following this suggestion, you will be approximating the time limits imposed by the board examinations previously mentioned.

When you have finished answering the questions in a chapter, you should then spend as much time as you need verifying your answers and carefully reading the explanations. Although you should pay special attention to the explanations for the questions you answered incorrectly, you should read every explanation. The explanations have been designed to reinforce and supplement the information tested by the questions. If, after reading the explanations for a given chapter, you feel you need still more information about the material covered, you should consult and study the references indicated.

This book meets the criteria established by the AMA's Department of Continuing Medical Education for up to 22 credit hours in Category 5D for the Physician's Recognition Award. It should provide an experience that is instructive as well as evaluative; we also hope that you enjoy it. We would be very happy to receive your comments.

Acknowledgement

As the editor of the third edition of *Obstetrics and Gynecology: Pre-Test Self-Assessment and Review;* I would like to express my gratitude to the editors of the previous editions. Many of their questions have been retained in principle with updates and modifications. Similarly, I wish to express my sincere appreciation to the McGraw-Hill Health Professions Division staff for their help in the preparation of this edition.

Mark I. Evans

BIOLOGY
AND PHYSIOLOGY
OF REPRODUCTION

Anatomy, Genetics, Embryology, and Congenital Anomalies

DIRECTIONS: Each question below contains five suggested answers. Choose the **one best** response to each question.

1. In a screening program for neural tube defects using maternal serum alpha-fetoprotein (MSAFP), the next step following two successive elevated MSAFP blood tests should be

(A) a third MSAFP
(B) ultrasound examination
(C) amniocentesis
(D) amniography
(E) recommendation of termination

2. The most important indication of surgical repair of a double uterus is

(A) habitual abortion
(B) dysmenorrhea
(C) menometrorrhagia
(D) dyspareunia
(E) premature delivery

3. The most common cause of ambiguous genitalia in infants is

(A) chromosomal nondisjunction
(B) gonadal dysgenesis
(C) adrenal hyperplasia
(D) mosaicism
(E) testicular feminization

4. The third trimester fetus of a mother with a balanced 13/13 translocation would have what likelihood of having an abnormal chromosome karyotype?

(A) 2 percent
(B) 10 percent
(C) 25 percent
(D) 50 percent
(E) 100 percent

5. Achondroplasia is best characterized by which of the following statements?

(A) The inheritance pattern is autosomal recessive
(B) Mutation accounts for 90 percent of all cases
(C) Cesarean section is rarely necessary
(D) Affected women rarely live to the reproductive age
(E) None of the above

6.   A 42-year-old woman undergoes a Marshall-Marchetti-Krantz operation for true urinary stress incontinence. The jack-knife position in which the knees are bent and abducted laterally is used during the procedure. Post-operatively, the patient complains of footdrop and loss of sensation on the dorsal apsect of her right foot. The nerve most likely to have been injured during this operation is the

(A) obturator
(B) internal pudendal
(C) common peroneal
(D) ilioinguinal
(E) genitofemoral

7.   The most common defect of the adrenogenital syndrome is

(A) idiopathic
(B) 11-hydroxylase deficiency
(C) 17-hydroxylase deficiency
(D) 21-hydroxylase deficiency
(E) 3-beta-ol-dehydrogenase deficiency

DIRECTIONS: Each question below contains four suggested answers of which **one or more** is correct. Choose the answer:

A	if	**1, 2, and 3**	are correct
B	if	**1 and 3**	are correct
C	if	**2 and 4**	are correct
D	if	**4**	is correct
E	if	**1, 2, 3, and 4**	are correct

8. The karyotypes associated with Turner syndrome include

(1) 46,XXr
(2) 46,XXp-
(3) 46,Xi(Xq)
(4) 46,X,i(Xp)

9. In patients with carcinoma of the vulva, lymphatic drainage characteristically

(1) is to the periaortic nodes
(2) is to the superficial inguinal lymph nodes
(3) bypasses the deep femoral lymph nodes
(4) is from the clitoral region to the deep femoral lymph nodes

10. The advantages of transverse abdominal incisions include

(1) a decreased incidence of incisional hernias
(2) the requirement of only light general anesthesia
(3) a scar that can be cosmetically hidden
(4) easy access to the upper abdomen for bowel surgery

11. A carrier of a balanced 14/21 (D/G) translocation is described by which of the following statements?

(1) Amniocentesis can detect offspring who have translocation Down syndrome as well as those who are balanced carriers
(2) Karyotype analysis would reveal 45 chromosomes in each cell
(3) Chromosome studies of members of a carrier's family are indicated to detect others at risk for having children with Down syndrome
(4) The risk for bearing children who have Down syndrome is the same whether the husband or the wife is the carrier

12. A group of congenital anomalies known collectively as Potter syndrome includes renal agenesis (or other renal anomalies) and pulmonary hypoplasia. Other anomalies associated with Potter syndrome include

(1) hydrocephaly
(2) amnion nodosum
(3) cleft palate
(4) oligohydramnios

13. Diseases that have a positive correlation between maternal infection during pregnancy and congenital anomalies in the fetus include

(1) rubella
(2) mumps
(3) cytomegalovirus
(4) influenza

14. Individuals with the karyotype 45,X are likely to have

(1) a webbed neck, shield chest, high-arched palate, and low-set ears
(2) lymphedema of the extremities at birth
(3) a high incidence of diabetes mellitus
(4) mothers who are over 35 years of age

15. True statements about a pregnant woman who has phenylketonuria include which of the following?

(1) If the father carries the gene, the risk that the child will be affected is 25 percent
(2) If the father carries the gene, amniocentesis and selective abortion can avert the birth of affected children
(3) Individuals with phenylketonuria rarely survive to the reproductive years
(4) Children born to mothers who have phenylketonuria are frequently mentally retarded

16. A bicornuate uterus (bicornis unicollis) is associated with

(1) failure of complete fusion of the müllerian duct system
(2) an increase in obstetrical complications
(3) an increase in urinary tract anomalies
(4) cervical and vaginal malformations

DIRECTIONS: The groups of questions below consist of lettered choices followed by several numbered items. For each numbered item select the **one** lettered choice with which it is **most** closely associated. Each lettered choice may be used once, more than once, or not at all.

Questions 17–19

For each situation below, select the appropriate inheritance pattern.

(A) Autosomal dominant
(B) Autosomal recessive
(C) X-linked recessive
(D) Codominant
(E) Multifactoral

17. G6PD deficiency

18. Neurofibromatosis

19. Haplotypes

Questions 20–24

For each structure that follows, select its embryological origin.

(A) Genital tubercle
(B) Genital swellings
(C) Urogenital sinus
(D) Urethral folds
(E) Müllerian ducts

20. Labia minora

21. Labia majora

22. Clitoris

23. Vagina

24. Fallopian tubes

Questions 25–29

Match the following female structures with their male homologues.

(A) Gubernaculum testis
(B) Prostate gland
(C) Scrotum
(D) Vas deferens
(E) Phallus

25. Paraurethral glands

26. Labia majora

27. Round ligament

28. Gartner's duct

29. Clitoris

Questions 30–34

For each description that follows, select the blood vessel with which it is most likely to be associated.

(A) Uterine vein
(B) Right ovarian vein
(C) Left ovarian vein
(D) Uterine artery
(E) Ovarian artery

30. Arises from the anterior branch of the hypogastric artery

31. Drains into the internal iliac veins

32. Drains into the inferior vena cava

33. Arises from the abdominal aorta

34. Drains into the left renal vein

Anatomy, Genetics, Embryology, and Congenital Anomalies

Answers

1. The answer is B. *(Gastel, p 43.)* The recommended sequence for a MSAFP screening program for 1000 hypothetical patients would have 50 with an elevated (2.5 multiples of the normal median) first MSAFP. About 30 would demonstrate elevated levels in the second MSAFP. Next, a thorough ultrasound exam should reveal about 15 patients with an obvious reason for the elevation: e.g., anencephaly, twins, wrong gestational age of fetus, or fetal demise. About 15 patients with no obvious cause should be offered amniocentesis. Of these 15 about 1 to 2 will have elevated amniotic fluid AFP confirmed by acetyl-cholinesterase. Such patients will have a greater than 99 percent chance of having a neural tube defect or other serious malformation. Amniography is an outmoded procedure in which radioopaque dye is injected into the amniotic cavity for the purpose of taking x-rays. Under no circumstances whatsoever should termination be recommended on the basis of MSAFP alone.

2. The answer is A. *(Mattingly, ed 5. pp 314–315.)* Habitual abortion is the most important indication for surgical treatment of women who have a double uterus. The abortion rate in women who have a double uterus is two to three times greater than that of the general population. Therefore, women who present with habitual abortion should be evaluated by hysterosalpingography to detect a possible double uterus. Dysmenorrhea, premature delivery, dyspareunia, and menometrorrhagia are other, less important indications for surgical intervention.

3. The answer is C. *(Thompson, ed 3. p 179.)* Although congenital adrenal hyperplasia affects both sexes, it more often is recognized in female infants. It accounts for approximately 50 percent of all cases of ambiguous sexual differentiation. Despite its genetic origin, congenital adrenal hyperplasia is not associated with karyotypic abnormalities. The most typical abnormality of external genitalia is clitoral enlargement, which is usually accompanied by some degree of hypospadias and labioscrotal fusion.

4. The answer is E. *(Thompson, ed 3. p 161.)* Carriers of balanced translocations of the same chromosome are phenotypically normal. However, in the process of gamete formation (either sperm or ova), the translocated chromosome cannot divide and therefore the meiosis products end up with either two copies or no copies of the particular chromosome. In the former case, fertilization leads to trisomy of that chromosome. Many trisomies are lethal in utero. Trisomies of 13, 18, and 21 lead to classic syndromes. In the latter case, a monosomy is produced, and all except for monosomy X (Turner syndrome) are lethal in utero.

5. The answer is B. *(Smith, ed 3. pp 248–251.)* Achondroplasia, a congenital disorder of cartilage formation characterized by dwarfism, is associated with an autosomal dominant pattern of inheritance. However, mutation accounts for 90 percent of all cases of the disorder. Affected women almost always require cesarean section because of the distorted shape of their pelves. Women who have achondroplasia and receive adequate treatment for its associated complications, including the neurological signs of cord compression due to spinal deformity, generally have a normal life expectancy.

6. The answer is C. *(Mattingly, ed 5. pp 33–36.)* The jack-knife position described in the question commonly gives rise to injury of the sciatic or peroneal nerve through the overstretching of the nerve over the sacrospinous ligament. The symptoms of footdrop and loss of sensation over the dorsal aspect of the foot classically accompany peroneal nerve injury. The ilioinguinal and genitofemoral nerves traverse the inguinal canal together with the round ligament. The obturator nerve, which runs along the lateral wall of the pelvis, can be damaged by deep retractors and during radical pelvic surgery. It supplies all of the adducter muscles of the thigh as well as provides the sensory supply to the medial aspects of the thigh. The internal pudendal nerve is derived from S_2-S_3 and supplies the vulva and perineum.

7. The answer is D. *(Speroff, ed 3. pp 344–345.)* This enzyme block is the most frequent cause of sexual ambiguity and the most frequent endocrine cause of neonatal death. Serum 17-hydroxyprogesterone and urinary pregnanetriol are elevated. Neonatal complications are related to salt loss because of inadequate mineralocorticoid production in some of these infants.

8.   The answer is A (1, 2, 3). *(Therman, pp 130–132.)* Although monosomy of the X chromosome (45,X) is the most common karyotype of patients who have Turner syndrome, a variety of structural abnormalities of the X chromosome in addition to mosaics may be found in patients who have this disorder. Comparison of chromosomal abnormalities and phenotypic features in individuals who have gonadal dysgenesis indicates that the short stature and other clinical findings of the Turner phenotype are associated with loss of the short arm of one X chromosome. Of the karyotypes listed in the question, all involve monosomy for a portion of the short arm of the X chromosome except 46,X,i(Xp). Individuals who have this karyotype have only one normal X chromosome; their other X chromosome, composed of a duplication of the normal short arm, is called an isochromosome. In essence, they are monosomic for the long arm of the X and trisomic for the short arm. This karyotype is associated with gonadal dysgenesis but not with the phenotypic features characteristic of individuals who have Turner syndrome.

9.   The answer is C (2, 4). *(Parsons, ed 2. p 1606.)* An important feature of the lymphatic drainage of the vulva is the existence of drainage across the midline. The vulva drains first into the superficial inguinal lymph nodes, then into the deep femoral nodes, and finally into the external iliac lymph nodes. The clinical significance of this sequence for patients with carcinoma of the vulva is that the iliac nodes are probably free of the disease if the deep femoral nodes are not involved. Unlike the lymphatic drainage from the rest of the vulva, the drainage from the clitoral region bypasses the superficial inguinal nodes and passes directly to the deep femoral nodes. Thus, while the superficial nodes will usually also have metastases when the deep femoral nodes are implicated, it is possible for only the deep nodes to be involved if the carcinoma is in the midline near the clitoris.

10.   The answer is B (1, 3). *(Mattingly, ed 5. pp 165–166.)* Benefits of a low transverse abdominal incision are a decreased incidence of incisional hernias and cosmetic placement of the scar near the edge of the pubic hairline. The use of light anesthesia is contraindicated because it provides poor muscle relaxation. Bowel surgery is best approached with a vertical incision, especially if a colostomy is anticipated.

11.   The answer is A (1, 2, 3). *(Thompson, ed 3. 148–150, 159–161, 348.)* Individuals who are carriers of a balanced D/G translocation have 45 chromosomes in each cell; one D-group and one G-group chromosome have fused, forming a chromosome that resembles a member of the C group. The risk for giving birth to children who have translocation Down syndrome is substantially higher if the wife is the carrier (10 to 12 percent) than if the husband is the carrier (2 to 3 percent). Amniocentesis can determine whether the offspring will be unaffected, will carry the translocation, or will have the disease. Because a D/G translocation can be inherited from a parent (approximately 50 percent are familial), chromosome studies of family members are recommended.

12. The answer is C (2, 4). *(Pritchard, ed 16. pp 577, 1000.)* An infant with Potter syndrome generally presents as a breech. After birth, the baby is never able to ventilate adequately. These infants rarely survive more than a few hours. The primary lesion in Potter syndrome is thought to be renal. Because of renal agenesis, urine output is impossible, and oligohydramnios results. Oligohydramnios is believed to lead to pulmonary hypoplasia, because lack of amniotic fluid somehow restricts normal lung development. The characteristic facial anomalies (large, low-set ears and flattened nose) are thought to be related to pressure on the face increased by a lack of cushioning amniotic fluid. The diagnosis of Potter syndrome has been made antenatally with the aid of ultrasonography. Demonstration of a fetal bladder that fills and empties should rule out Potter syndrome. The absence of evidence of a bladder, despite repeated ultrasonographic examinations, would be compatible with the diagnosis. Amnion nodosum, another common finding in Potter syndrome, consists of multiple opaque nodules in the amnion. Their etiology is not clear, but they represent fetal squames that have become "parasitic" on the membranes.

13. The answer is B (1, 3). *(Burrow, ed 2. pp 333–350.)* Rubella syndrome in the newborn secondary to rubella infection during pregnancy (especially, not exclusively, during the first trimester) is well known. Although cytomegalovirus infection is less familiar, it is thought to cause congenital anomalies in about 500 newborns every year in the United States. The abnormalities are usually in the central nervous system and include microcephaly, cerebral calcifications, deafness, and other mental and motor disabilities. Although there have been some suggestions that influenza epidemics have led to a subsequent rise in the incidence of childhood leukemia, this relationship has not been established; in fact, there is no proof that influenza is associated with any anomalies. Mumps is relatively common during pregnancy, but prospective studies have failed to show any associated congenital anomalies.

14. The answer is A (1, 2, 3). *(Smith, ed 3. pp 72–75.)* Individuals with a 45,X karyotype have Turner's syndrome (gonadal dysgenesis), a disorder in phenotypic females characterized by a variety of physical abnormalities. In addition to those listed in the questions, pigmented nevi, a short fourth metacarpal, wide-set nipples, and renal and cardiovascular anomalies are common. Lymphedema presents as puffiness of the hands and feet at birth. Diabetes mellitus is also prevalent among these children. Gonadal dysgenesis, unlike other chromosomal abnormalities, is not related to maternal age.

15. The answer is D (4). *(Smith, ed 3. p 434.)* If a woman who has phenylketonuria (PKU), which is an autosomal recessive disorder, marries a carrier for this disease, the chance that offspring will be affected is 50 percent. Although phenylketonuria cannot be detected prenatally, screening of newborns and early institution of low-phenylalanine diets have made it possible for affected individuals to reach adulthood. It has become apparent that high frequency of mental redardation exists in children of mothers who have phenylketonuria, even if these children do not themselves have the disease. Retardation in these children presumably is related to intrauterine exposure to high phenylalanine levels in the maternal blood. Whether or not a PKU mother can be "compelled" to follow a diet for the sake of the developing fetus will be a significant ethical debate of the late 1980's.

16. The answer is A (1, 2, 3). *(Parsons, ed 2. pp 683–686.)* Failure of fusion of the müllerian ducts can give rise to the several types of uterine anomalies of which uterus bicornis unicollis is a representative type. This condition is associated with higher obstetrical complications, such as an increase in the rate of second trimester abortion and premature labor. If the pregnancies go to term, malpresentations such as breech and transverse lies are frequent. Also, prolonged labor, which is probably due to inadequate muscle development in the uterus, increased bleeding, and a higher incidence of fetal anomalies caused by defective implantation of the placenta all occur far more commonly than in normal pregnancies. An intravenous pyelogram is mandatory in the workup of patients with uterine anomalies as there is an associated higher incidence of urinary tract anomalies. In uterus bicornis unicollis, there is a single cervix with a normal vagina.

17–19. The answers are: 17-C, 18-A, 19-D *(Thompson, ed 3. pp 114, 190–197. Smith, ed 3. pp 377–379.)* Glucose-6-phosphate dehydrogenase deficiency is X-linked recessive and is found predominantly in males of African and Mediterranean origin. Although the causes of clinical manifestations in G6PD are multifactorial (e.g., sulfa drugs) the inheritance is not. Neurofibromatosis, whose occurrance is often sporadic (i.e., a spontaneous mutation in 50 percent) is inherited as an autosomal dominant once the gene is in a family. The severity of the condition can be very variable even within the same family. The HLA antigens (four from each parent) are all expressed and therefore do not show any "dominance" in their expression. Certain combinations of haplotypes are associated with some disease conditions (such as 21-hydroxylase deficiency congential adrenal hyperplasia) in that they occur much more commonly than would be expected by chance; however, such associations do not, alone, define inheritance.

20–24. The answers are: 20-D, 21-B, 22-A, 23-C, 24-E. *(Green, ed 3. pp 77–80, 88–96, 103, 109.)* In the female, the urethral folds give rise to the labia minora, while the labia majora are formed from the genital swellings. It is believed that the development of external genitalia is dependent on the presence of hormones during the intrauterine period. With the absence of androgens and the inducer substance in females, the wolffian duct system regresses while the external genitalia develop under the influence of estrogen from both maternal and placental sources.

In the male, the genital tubercle gives rise to the phallus, while in the female it elongates minimally to form the clitoris. Clitoral hypertrophy can occur in conditions where there is an abnormally high level of circulating androgens during the critical phase of development of the external genitalia. Congenital adrenal hyperplasia and mixed gonadal dysgenesis are two clinical situations that may present with clitoral hypertrophy.

There are several theories to explain the embryological origin of the vagina; however it is generally accepted that the upper two-thirds of the vagina are of müllerian duct origin while the lower one-third is of urogenital sinus origin, which seems to explain in part the congenital anomalies that arise in this anatomical region. A common anomaly of urogenital sinus origin is imperforate hymen, which is easily treated by hymenotomy. Congenital absence of the vagina is an anomaly of mullerian duct origin and, as such, usually involves an absence of only the upper two-thirds of the vagina, as well as an absence of the uterus and fallopian tubes in most cases.

In the female, the müllerian ducts give rise to the fallopian tubes, uterus, and cervix. Imperfect fusion of the müllerian ducts can give rise to a whole spectrum of uterine anomalies, which may be associated with clinical entities like habitual abortions, prematurity, and fetal malpositions. Patients with proven müllerian duct anomalies should have an intraveous pyelogram to rule out urinary tract anomalies that may be present.

25–29. The answers are: 25-B, 26-C, 27-A, 28-D, 29-E. *(Novak, ed 9. pp 1–3, 438.)* The male homologue of the round ligament is the gubernacluum testis. It is a cordlike structure extending from the lower pole of the testis to the scrotum. Abnormalities of this structure are associated with maldescent of the testes. The round ligaments play a minor role in support of the uterus.

The prostate gland corresponds with the paraurethral glands in females. Clinically, these glands and their canals, which open into both the urethra and the Skene's ducts, can serve as a reservoir for gonococcal infections. Also these glands can become cystic with chronic infections, giving rise to suburethral diverticula.

In the embryological development of the external genitalia of the female, the urethral folds and the genital swellings do not fuse, giving rise to the labia minora and the labia majora, respectively. The contrary is true in the male, as the urethral folds fuse to form the penis, while the scrotum is formed by the fusion of the genital swellings.

The vas deferens and Gartner's duct are both derived from the wolffian duct system. Cysts of Gartner's duct, when present, are usually found along the anterolateral wall of the vagina. They are usually asymptomatic and rarely require surgical intervention.

Embryologically, the male phallus and the female clitoris both arise from the genital tubercle. Hypertrophy of the clitoris can occur if there is a high level of androgens present during the early development of the external genitalia.

30–34. The answers are: 30-D, 31-A, 32-B, 33-E, 34-C. *(Mattingly, ed 5. pp 36–38.)* The blood supply of the pelvic organs and musculature is derived primarily from the hypogastric artery. The uterine artery arises from the anterior division of the hypogastric artery and supplies the vagina, uterus, and fallopian tubes. The bladder is also supplied by the vesical branches of the hypogastric artery, which terminates as the internal pudendal artery supplying the perineum, labia, and clitoris, as well as the thigh muscles. The uterine veins, which drain into the internal iliac veins, generally follow the course of the uterine arteries. Together, they course superiorly to the ureters along the base of the broad ligaments.

The two ovarian veins follow different courses. The right ovarian vein drains into the inferior vena cava just below the level of the right renal vein, while the left ovarian vein drains into the left renal vein. The right ovarian vein may become distended during pregnancy, causing partial obstruction of the ureter proximal to its course. This has been postulated to be a cause of right hydronephrosis in pregnancy. The ovarian artery arises from the abdominal aorta. It courses through the infundibulopelvic ligament and supplies the ovary and the fallopian tube.

A thorough understanding of the above-mentioned relationships is essential in gynecological surgery, especially in cases of hemorrhage requiring hypogastric artery ligation.

Puberty, Menstruation, Menopause, Sexuality, and Conception

DIRECTIONS: Each question below contains five suggested answers. Choose the **one best** response to each question.

35. Follicle-stimulating hormone is elaborated by

(A) chromophobe cells of the adenohypophysis
(B) basophilic cells of the adenohypophysis
(C) acidophilic cells of the adenohypophysis
(D) theca interna cells
(E) all of the above

36. In what percentage of girls with precocious puberty is this constitutional (nonorganic) in origin?

(A) 10 percent
(B) 25 percent
(C) 30 percent
(D) 50 percent
(E) 90 percent

37. Peripheral conversion of estrogen precursors in the obese patient after menopause results primarily in the formation of

(A) estriol
(B) estradiol
(C) estrone
(D) androstenedione
(E) dehydroepiandrosterone

38. The ovaries of an infant at birth contain oocytes that have progressed to

(A) prophase of the first meiotic division
(B) formation of oogonia
(C) maturation
(D) anaphase of the second meiotic division
(E) none of the above

39. In the testis, which of the following can be *directly* influenced by luteinizing hormone (LH)?

(A) Leydig cells
(B) Sertoli cells
(C) Leydig cells and Sertoli cells
(D) Leydig cells and seminiferous tubules
(E) Sertoli cells and seminferous tubules

40. Which of the following allows for the *earliest* determination of probable pregnancy?

(A) Pelvic examination
(B) Ultrasonography
(C) Basal temperature curves
(D) Hemagglutination-inhibition test
(E) Assay of the serum beta subunit of human chorionic gonadotropin

41. If a man received a severe thermal trauma to his testes, his previously normal sperm count would become depressed in about

(A) 1 day
(B) 7 days
(C) 30 days
(D) 75 days
(E) 100 days

42. The average blood loss resulting from menstruation is

(A) 10 to 15 ml
(B) 25 to 50 ml
(C) 75 to 100 ml
(D) 101 to 125 ml
(E) 130 to 150 ml

43. According to Masters and Johnson, factors that increase the likelihood of female orgasm during intercourse include

(A) a larger clitoral glans
(B) a clitoris located closer to the vaginal introitus
(C) erection of the clitoral shaft
(D) male superior coital position
(E) none of the above

44. All of the following steps in the mechanism of action of adrenocortico-tropic hormone (ACTH) are correct EXCEPT that

(A) ACTH is bound by specific surface receptors on the adrenal cortical cell
(B) in the presence of magnesium, adenylcyclase is activated and the intracellular concentration of adenosine 3':5'-cyclic phosphate (cyclic AMP) increases
(C) cyclic AMP phosphorylates key enzymes
(D) key enzymes facilitate the conversion of cholesterol to pregnenolone
(E) synthesis of new proteins occurs and increases adrenal weight

DIRECTIONS: Each question below contains four suggested answers of which **one or more** is correct. Choose the answer:

A	if	**1, 2, and 3**	are correct
B	if	**1 and 3**	are correct
C	if	**2 and 4**	are correct
D	if	**4**	is correct
E	if	**1, 2, 3, and 4**	are correct

45. Vaginismus is

(1) a reflex spastic involuntary contraction of the vaginal outlet
(2) detectable on pelvic examination
(3) associated with secondary impotence in the male partner
(4) in part treated with vaginal dilators

46. Physiological processes that are estrogen-dependent in women include which of the following?

(1) Menses
(2) Vaginal cornification
(3) Appearance of axillary hair
(4) Cervical mucus formation

47. The menopause invariably is accompanied by

(1) osteoporosis
(2) anxiety and depression
(3) cardiovascular degeneration
(4) decreased serum estrogen levels

48. Sequelae of vasectomy include

(1) varicocele
(2) sperm granuloma
(3) torsion of the testis
(4) the production of sperm antibodies

49. Waning estrogen levels in perimenopausal women can produce which of the following responses?

(1) Vasomotor instability
(2) Atrophic vaginitis
(3) Decreased libido
(4) Osteoporosis

50. Significant components of vaginal lubrication include

(1) fluid from Skene's glands
(2) mucus produced by endocervical glands
(3) viscous fluid from Bartholin's glands
(4) transudatelike material from the vaginal walls

51. Physiological actions occurring during the plateau phase of sexual excitement in women include

(1) areolar tumescence
(2) systolic blood pressure elevations
(3) involuntary skeletal muscle contractions
(4) involuntary contractions of the rectal sphincter

SUMMARY OF DIRECTIONS

A	B	C	D	E
1,2,3 only	1,3 only	2,4 only	4 only	All are correct

52. Characteristics of the gonadotropins (FSH and LH) include

(1) stimulation of the production of primordial follicles
(2) stimulation of the production of estrogen by thecal cells
(3) stimulation of the production of spermatozoa and testosterone in men who have hypopituitarism
(4) a glycoprotein structure

53. Rising estradiol levels can have which of the following hormonal effects?

(1) Suppression of LH
(2) Stimulation of LH
(3) Suppression of FSH
(4) Stimulation of FSH

54. The luteal phase of the menstrual cycle primarily involves

(1) the Δ^4-3-ketone pathway
(2) the Δ^5-3β-hydroxy pathway
(3) granulosa cells
(4) theca cells

55. The contraceptive effect of birth control pills containing both synthetic estrogen and progestin is related to the

(1) inhibition of ovulation
(2) impaired penetrability of sperm into the cervical mucus
(3) atrophic changes of the endometrium impairing implantation
(4) uterotubal hypermotility impairing sperm transport

56. True statements about sexual activity in late pregnancy include which of the following?

(1) Intercourse during the third trimester can lead to premature labor
(2) Intercourse during the third trimester can promote premature rupture of membranes and intrauterine infection
(3) Prostaglandins in semen have been shown to contribute to the initiation of labor
(4) Orgasm is contraindicated in women who have a history of premature labor

57. Cholesterol can be synthesized from acetate by which of the following organs?

(1) Ovary
(2) Adrenal gland
(3) Testis
(4) Placenta

58. Polypeptide structure and direct inducement of hormonal changes in target organs are characteristics of which of the following hormones?

(1) Prolactin
(2) Growth hormone
(3) Chorionic somatomammotropin
(4) Thyrotropin

DIRECTIONS: The groups of questions below consist of lettered choices followed by several numbered items. For each numbered item select the **one** lettered choice with which it is **most** closely associated. Each lettered choice may be used once, more than once, or not at all.

Questions 59–63
Match each action listed below with the appropriate enzyme.

(A) Adenylcyclase
(B) 5 α-Reductase
(C) 17β-Hydroxylase
(D) 20-Hydroxylase
(E) 21-Dehydroxylase

59. Is activated by LH

60. Converts androstenedione to testosterone

61. Converts testosterone to dihydro-testosterone

62. Catalyzes the first step in the production of hormonal steroids from cholesterol

63. Causes massive adrenal enlargement when congenitally deficient, is associated with poor survival of the affected infants, and can lead to the formation of female genitalia in genotypically male infants

Puberty, Menstruation, Menopause, Sexuality, and Conception

Answers

35. The answer is B. *(Jones, ed 10. p 47.)* Luteinizing hormone (LH) and follicle-stimulating hormone (FSH) are synthesized, stored, and secreted from the basophilic cells of the anterior pituitary. It appears that a single cell type makes both LH and FSH.

36. The answer is E. *(Speroff, ed 3. pp 370–374.)* In constitutional sexual precocity there is premature maturation of the hypothalamic-pituitary-ovarian axis, resulting in production of gonadotropins and sex steroids. This is usually a diagnosis of exclusion and deserves long-term follow-up for detection of possible organic problems.

37. The answer is C. *(Speroff, ed 3. p 110.)* The circulating level of estrone in the postmenopausal woman is higher than that of estradiol. Estrone is principally derived from peripheral conversion of androstenedione in adipose tissue. The percent conversion of androstenedione to estrogen correlates with body weight.

38. The answer is A. *(Speroff, ed 3. p 103.)* Evidence of nuclear maturation is first seen at about 15 weeks of gestation. The oogonia are transformed to oocytes as they enter the first meiotic division and arrest in prophase. The second meiotic division is not completed until fertilization.

39. The answer is A. *(Williams, ed 6. pp 296–303.)* In the testis, Leydig cells produce testosterone, Sertoli cells primarily provide structural support and nutrition, and seminiferous tubules produce sperm. Leydig cells are under the influence of luteinizing hormone (LH) in a negative-feedback relationship. Testosterone produced by Leydig cells regulates spermatogenesis; therefore, seminiferous tubules are indirectly affected by LH secretion.

40. The answer is E. *(Speroff, ed 3. pp 285–286.)* Human chorionic gonadotropin (HCG) supports the corpus luteum of early pregnancy and can be first detected in maternal blood on about the eighth day after ovulation. This is well before a sustained rise in basal body temperature. Pelvic examination and ultrasonography do not generally detect pregnancy until about the fourth week after ovulation.

41. The answer is D. *(Speroff, ed 3. p 510.)* Severe thermal trauma to the testes, such as that caused by extremes of cold or heat, can inhibit the development of sperm. Depression in the sperm count usually appears in about 75 days, the length of time in which an immature spermatid develops into a spermatozoon. Either oligospermia or azoospermia can result.

42. The answer is B. *(Speroff, ed 3. p 233.)* The normal volume of menstrual blood loss is about 30 ml. A volume greater than 100 ml is considered abnormal.

43. The answer is E. *(Masters, 1966. pp 48, 56–59.)* Masters and Johnson have shown that the size of the clitoris bears no relation to increased orgasmic capacity. Similarly, the distance between the clitoris and the vaginal introitus makes little difference, because clitoral stimulation during coition is provided largely by traction on the clitoral hood via the labia minora, which are moved during penile thrusting. Direct clitoral stimulation can be achieved only by the lateral and female superior coital positions. Erection of the clitoris is likewise not related to orgasmic capacity.

44. The answer is B. *(Williams, ed 6. p 79.)* Adrenocorticotropic hormone (ACTH) binds to specific cell-surface receptors in the adrenal cortex and is concentrated from the plasma. The combined action of ACTH and calcium stimulates adenylcyclase to catalyze production of adenosine 3':5'-cyclic phosphate (cyclic AMP), which in turn causes enzyme phosphorylation. These enzymes convert precursors to active hormones; cholesterol, for example, is converted enzymatically to pregnenolone. Cyclic AMP also induces synthesis of RNA, which in turn stimulates protein synthesis; as a result, adrenal weight is increased.

45. The answer is E (all). *(Kase, pp 505–506, 975.)* Vaginismus is painful spasm of the pelvic muscles and vaginal outlet and is usually psychogenic. It should be differentiated from frigidity, which implies lack of sexual desire. Treatment is primarily psychotherapeutic as organic causes are very rare.

46. The answer is E (all). *(Speroff, ed 3. pp 70–71.)* The presence of estrogen in a pubertal woman stimulates the formation of secondary sex characteristics, including development of breasts, appearance of axillary hair, production of cervical mucus, and vaginal cornification. As estrogen levels increase, menses begins and ovulation is maintained for several decades. Decreasing levels of estrogen lower the frequency of ovulation, eventually leading to the menopause.

47. The answer is D (4). *(Kase, pp 337–338, 342.)* The sine qua non of the menopause is ovarian failure; a marked decrease in estrogen production subsequently results, and a secondary increase in the production of FSH by the pituitary is noted. Symptoms of emotional upset may be due more to a change in life situation than to a change in hormonal balance. Cardiovascular and bony degeneration occurs in some, but by no means all, women. Estrogen replacement therapy should probably be limited to women with climacteric symptoms because recent data suggest that estrogen use by postmenopausal women may be associated with the development of endometrial carcinoma; its use is least effective in treating women who develop osteoporosis.

48. The answer is C (2, 4). *(Sciarra, ed 2, vol 6, chap 47. pp 7–11.)* Vasectomy involves division of each ductus deferens via a scrotal incision. There is no demonstrable effect on androgen production, libido, or sexual performance. Granuloma formation occasionally follows, but is not a serious clinical problem. There have been some reports of antibody production to sperm after vasectomy.

49. The answer is E (all). *(Speroff, ed 3. pp 116–125.)* In menopausal and postmenopausal women, waning estrogen levels can produce atrophic vaginitis, decreased libido, vasomotor instability, osteoporosis, and psychological symptoms (including depression and anxiety). Vasomotor instability causes the familiar hot flashes of menopausal women. These responses may be due to an unstable relationship, caused by decreased estrogen levels, between the autonomic nervous system and the hypothalamus.

50. The answer is D (4). *(Masters, 1966. p 69.)* Masters and Johnson observed a transudatelike fluid emanating directly from the vaginal walls during sexual response. This mucoid material, which is sufficient for complete vaginal lubrication, is produced by transudation from the venous plexus surrounding the vagina and appears seconds after the initiation of sexual excitement. No activity by Skene's glands was noted, and production of cervical mucus during sexual stimulation was observed in only a very few subjects. Fluid from Batholin's glands appears long after vaginal lubrication is well established; it may, however, make a minor contribution to lubrication in the late plateau phase.

51. The answer is A (1, 2, 3). *(Masters, 1966. pp 27–37.)* The response of women to sexual stimulation is generalized and affects many different organ systems. Physiological responses include superficial and deep vasocongestion accounting for, among other things, enlargement and changes of color of extragenital and genital areas. Voluntary and involuntary myotonia, both generalized and specific, also may occur, although involuntary contractions of the rectal sphincter are usually detected only during the orgasmic phase.

52. The answer is E (all). *(Williams, ed 6. pp 81–83.)* The gonadotropins (FSH and LH) are glycoproteins. In women, they stimulate the production of one or more primordial follicles and induce thecal cells in the ovary to produce estrogen. In a man who has hypopituitarism, the gonadotropins can cause production of spermatozoa and testosterone.

53. The answer is A (1, 2, 3). *(Speroff, ed 3. pp 84–86.)* Estradiol has a negative-feedback relationship with FSH and both a negative-feedback and a positive-feedback relationship with LH. Rising estradiol levels suppress the production of FSH and LH. As estradiol levels continue to increase, however, LH levels begin to rise. Negative feedback (suppression of LH and FSH production) is mediated by estradiol effects on the hypothalamus and pituitary gland; positive feedback (increase in LH) also is controlled by the hypothalamic centers.

54. The answer is B (1, 3). *(Speroff, ed 3. pp 9–12.)* In the luteal phase of the menstrual cycle, granulosa cells produce estrogen by way of the Δ^4-3-ketone pathway, in which progesterone is a precursor. Theca cells in the follicular phase of the menstrual cycle manufacture estrogen by the Δ^5-3β-hydroxy pathway; pregnenolone, dehydroepiandrosterone, and estradiol – but not progesterone – are essential precursors of this pathway.

55. The answer is A (1, 2, 3). *(Kase, p 1010.)* The marked effectiveness of the combined oral contraceptive pill, which contains a synthetic estrogen and a progestin, is related to its multiple antifertility actions. The primary effect is to suppress gonadotropins, thus inhibiting ovulation. The prolonged progestational effect also causes thickening of the cervical mucus and atrophic changes of the endometrium, thus impairing sperm penetrability and ovum implantation, respectively.

56. The answer is D (4). *(Sciarra, ed 2, vol 6, chap 100, p 3.)* Several clinical surveys have failed to reveal any firm association between intercourse and premature labor, premature rupture of membranes, or intrauterine infection. On the other hand, orgasm, regardless of how it is achieved, can be harmful to women who have a history of premature delivery or a prematurely ripe cervix, because of accompanying uterine contractions. A fetal head that is engaged in the pelvis may be bumped during coitus; although this may frighten the parents, no demonstrable harm to the infant results. The physiological role of prostaglandins in human semen is unknown.

57. The answer is A (1, 2, 3). *(Speroff, ed 3. p 7.)* The conversion of acetate to cholesterol and, hence, to all the other steroid hormones can occur in the ovary, testis, and adrenal gland. The placenta, however, lacks the essential enzyme systems to perform this synthesis. Therefore, cholesterol, the basic building block in the synthesis of steroid hormones, must be supplied to the placenta. The fetus and the mother supply the cholesterol essential for steroidogenesis in the placenta. It has been suggested that the maternal cholesterol serves as the precursor for progesterone production, while fetal cholesterol is used for estrogen production.

58. The answer is A (1, 2, 3). *(Williams, ed 6. p 84.)* Growth hormone and chorionic somatomammotropin are polypeptide hormones composed of 191 amino-acid subunits, of which 161 are identical (the other 30 are closely related and vary by only a simple base change in the DNA template). Although the structure of human prolactin is not yet clearly established, it too is a polypeptide hormone of close to 200 subunits, many of which are in the same sequence as the other two hormones. Prolactin, growth hormone, and chorionic somatomammotropin are all able to induce hormonal changes directly in their target organs. Thyrotropin is a glycoprotein; its only physiological action is stimulation of the thyroid gland to produce another hormone, thyroxine, which is the mediator of thyroid activity.

59-63. The answers are: 59-A, 60-C, 61-B, 62-D, 63-D. *(Williams, ed 6. pp 285–286, 296–303.)* Testosterone reaching a target organ, such as the prostate gland, is converted to dihydrotestosterone by 5α-reductase, an enzyme in the cell wall or cell membrane. Adenylcyclase, which is an intracellular enzyme activated by the presence of LH, catalyzes the formation of cyclic AMP, which then activates other intracellular enzyme reactions. The enzyme 17β-hydroxylase is found primarily in the testis but also in the adrenal gland; it converts androstenedione to testosterone by hydroxylating the 17 position.

The conversion of cholesterol into steroid hormones begins with hydroxylation at the 30 position followed by cleavage of the six-carbon side chain (carbons 22 to 27); both reactions, which result in production of pregnenolone, are catalyzed by 20-hydroxylase (also known as cholesterol desmolase). Congenital deficiencies of this enzyme can cause the adrenal glands to fill with cholesterol and become greatly enlarged; affected infants, some of whom may be phenotypic females but genotypic males, have a poor prognosis.

Pregnancy, Lactation, and Puerperium

DIRECTIONS: Each question below contains five suggested answers. Choose the **one best** response to each question.

64. The earliest diagnosis of pregnancy by a sensitive serum BHCG assay is possible

(A) 1 hour after implantation
(B) during the week before the anticipated menses
(C) the day of anticipated menses
(D) 1 week following the missed menses

65. During pregnancy a woman needs additional iron to satisfy the demands of the fetus, the placenta, and her own increasing hemoglobin mass. The total antepartum iron need is approximately

(A) 250 mg
(B) 800 mg
(C) 1350 mg
(D) 1900 mg
(E) none of the above

66. All of the following statements about the endometrial Arias-Stella reaction in pregnant women are true EXCEPT that

(A) it was first described in association with tubal pregnancy
(B) it is a reaction of glandular epithelial cells
(C) it is a sign of impending fetal death
(D) affected cells have abundant, eosinophilic-staining cytoplasm
(E) the nuclei of affected cells are hyperchromatic and increased in size

67. An elevation of prolactin levels is caused by all the following physiological states EXCEPT

(A) sleep
(B) stress
(C) exercise
(D) parturition
(E) puerperium

68. Which of the following statements best characterizes the estrogen present in maternal urine?

(A) Its concentration is decreased during pregnancy
(B) It is 80 to 85 percent estriol at term
(C) It is 50 percent estradiol at term
(D) Its excretion is normal at term in patients who have placental sulfatase deficiency
(E) Its excretion is unrelated to fetal adrenal or hepatic function

69. All of the following statements about renal function in normal pregnancy are true EXCEPT that

(A) caliceal, renal pelvic, and ureteral dilatation can occur as early as the second trimester
(B) hormonal and mechanical factors have been implicated as causes of ureteral dilatation in the third trimester
(C) glomerular filtration rate increases about 50 percent over values in nonpregnant women
(D) renal plasma flow increases about 35 percent over values in nonpregnant women
(E) creatinine clearance is an accurate reflection of glomerular filtration rate during pregnancy

70. At 12 weeks gestation, amniotic fluid volume is approximately

(A) 50 ml
(B) 100 ml
(C) 150 ml
(D) 200 ml
(E) 250 ml

71. The maximum amniotic fluid volume is usually reached at what gestational age?

(A) 32 to 34 weeks
(B) 34 to 36 weeks
(C) 36 to 38 weeks
(D) 38 to 40 weeks
(E) 40 to 42 weeks

72. As pregnancy progresses, which of the following hematological changes occurs?

(A) Plasma volume increases proportionally more than red-cell volume
(B) Red-cell volume increases proportionally more than plasma volume
(C) Plasma volume increases and red-cell volume remains constant
(D) Red-cell volume decreases and plasma volume remains constant
(E) Neither plasma volume nor red-cell volume changes

73. The maternal mortality rate refers to the number of maternal deaths that occur as the result of the reproductive process per

(A) 1000 births
(B) 10,000 births
(C) 100,000 births
(D) 10,000 live births
(E) 100,000 live births

74. A 23-year-old woman (gravida 2, para 2) calls her physician 7 days post-partum because she is concerned that she is still bleeding from the vagina. It would be appropriate to tell this woman that it is normal for bloody lochia to last up to

(A) 2 days
(B) 5 days
(C) 8 days
(D) 11 days
(E) 14 days

75. During the first postpartum week, the uterus will lose what percent of its immediate postpartum weight?

(A) 10 percent
(B) 30 percent
(C) 50 percent
(D) 70 percent
(E) 90 percent

DIRECTIONS: Each question below contains four suggested answers of which **one or more** is correct. Choose the answer:

A	if	**1, 2, and 3**	are correct
B	if	**1 and 3**	are correct
C	if	**2 and 4**	are correct
D	if	**4**	is correct
E	if	**1, 2, 3, and 4**	are correct

76. Changes in the respiratory system during pregnancy include

(1) increased tidal volume
(2) decreased residual volume
(3) increased respiratory minute volume
(4) increased respiratory rate

77. Which of the following physiological changes can occur during a normal pregnancy?

(1) Decrease in fasting blood β-hydroxybutyric acid
(2) Increase in postprandial blood glucose
(3) Increase in fasting blood glucose
(4) Increase in postprandial insulin

78. Which of the following thyroxine-related changes can occur during pregnancy?

(1) Increase of total serum thyroxine
(2) Increase of free thyroxine
(3) Increase of thyroxine-binding globulin
(4) Decrease of thyroid-stimulating hormone

79. Which of the following laboratory values can be expected to increase during pregnancy?

(1) Serum albumin
(2) Plasma fibrinogen
(3) Blood urea nitrogen
(4) Erythrocyte sedimentation rate

80. Pregnancy can be considered diabetogenic because elevated levels of which of the following substances increase insulin secretion?

(1) Progesterone
(2) Estrogen
(3) Growth hormone
(4) Human chorionic sommatomammotropin

81. Urinary estriol levels can decrease in women taking

(1) methenamine mandelate (Mandelamine)
(2) ampicillin
(3) corticosteroids
(4) phenolphthalein cathartics

82. Breast cancer

(1) cannot be safely diagnosed by mammogram in pregnancy
(2) may mimic benign mastitis in pregnancy
(3) is a contraindication for future pregnancy
(4) in the first and second trimester of pregnancy should be treated the same as in the nonpregnant patient

83. Following delivery

(1) Menstruation may resume by 6 to 8 weeks in most nonlactating women
(2) approximately one-third of lactating women will resume menses by 3 months
(3) ovulation may occur within 6 weeks in lactating women
(4) women treated with bromocryptine for lactation suppression may ovulate by the second postpartum week

84. In the mother, suckling leads to which of the following responses?

(1) Release of oxytocin
(2) Decrease of prolactin inhibitory factor
(3) Decrease of hypothalamic dopamine
(4) Increase of luteinizing-hormone releasing factor

85. Of the following statements, which is/are true?

(1) There are no predictive factors for a patient at high risk for developing postpartum depression
(2) Prenatal preventive intervention for patients at high risk for postpartum depression is best managed alone by a mental health professional
(3) Postpartum depression is a self-limiting process that lasts for a maximum of 3 months
(4) About 10 to 12 percent of women develop postpartum depression

Pregnancy, Lactation
and Puerperium

Answers

64. The answer is B. *(Danforth ed 4. p 343. Speroff, ed 3. p 286.)* Sensitive assays use radioimmunoassay, which employs antibodies specific to the βsubunit of HCG. Many assays use a cutoff point of approximately 35 mIU/ml. βHCG can be demonstrated on the ninth day past the midcycle gonadotropin surge, which corresponds to 8 days past ovulation and 1 day following implantation.

65. The answer is B. *(Pritchard, ed 16. pp 234–235.)* The fetus and placenta contain approximately 300 mg of elemental iron at birth. In addition, the maternal increase in hemoglobin mass accounts for about 500 mg of elemental iron. Thus, the total antepartum iron requirement is 800 mg. Most of this iron is needed during the second half of pregnancy, at an approximate rate of 5.7 mg daily during the last 140 days. However, because about 1 mg of iron is excreted daily, the total daily iron need is almost 7 mg during the second half of pregnancy. Most women of childbearing age cannot mobilize this much iron, and supplemental iron must be given to prevent iron deficiency. The usual iron supplement, ferrous sulfate, contains 20 percent elemental iron. Thus, a 325 mg tablet contains about 65 mg of elemental iron, of which 10 to 20 percent will be absorbed. Most prenatal vitamins contain 60 or 65 mg of iron, and these should be adequate for a healthy pregnant woman. If iron stores have been depleted by poor dietary habits, recent childbirth, or other causes, however, additional iron supplementation may be necessary.

66. The answer is C. *(Mattingly, ed 5. p 372.)* Although the Arias-Stella reaction was first described in association with tubal pregnancy, it can occur in association with any condition in which active chorial tissue is present; these conditions include abortions, syncytial endometritis, hydatidiform mole, and choriocarcinoma. The Arias-Stella reaction affects glandular epithelial cells of the endometrium. These cells have abundant, vacuolated, eosinophilic cytoplasm and enlarged, hyperchromatic nuclei. This endometrial-gland reaction occurs after fetal death.

67. The answer is E. *(Yen, pp 158–165.)* Prolactin is released episodically in humans, with the highest levels being recorded during the nocturnal sleeping hours and the lowest levels during the waking hours of 10 a.m. to 12 a.m. Several other physiological stimuli, such as the stress of anesthesia, surgery, and exercise, have been shown to cause a rise in prolactin levels. In women, prolactin levels start to rise during the first trimester of pregnancy to a concentration ten times greater than that of the nonpregnant state. In the puerperium, prolactin levels decrease, reaching the normal range by the second or third week after delivery.

68. The answer is B. *(Aladjem, ed 2. pp 262–266.)* Total urinary estrogens at term are markedly elevated when compared to those of a nonpregnant woman. Estriol constitutes 80 to 85 percent of this urinary estrogen; its precursors are derived from the fetal liver and adrenal glands. When placental sulfatase activity is diminished, urinary excretion of estriol markedly decreases.

69. The answer is E. *(Aladjem, ed 2. pp 15–17, 23.)* Controlled studies have shown that, during pregnancy, creatinine clearance can vary by ± 50 percent when compared to inulin clearance, the accepted measure of glomerular filtration rate. A higher level of plasma creatinine results in tubular excretion; as a consequence, clearance by the kidney appears to be elevated. Creatinine clearance gives an accurate estimate of glomerular filtration rate only when the latter is less than 20 ml/min.

70. The answer is A. *(Pritchard, ed 16. pp 206, 603.)* At 12 weeks gestation, amniotic fluid volume is approximately 50 ml, rapidly increasing to about 200 ml by 16 weeks. For this reason, pregnancy termination by intraamniotic instillation of saline or prostaglandin solutions is extremely difficult at 12 weeks but becomes relatively simple beyond 16 weeks. Some authorities believe that termination by suction abortion is dangerous beyond 12 weeks, and that the month between 12 and 16 weeks is a time when no method is safe. More recently, however, several studies have indicated that surgical abortion through the vagina is safe up to at least 16 weeks gestation.

71. The answer is C. *(Pritchard, ed 16. pp 206–208.)* The maximum amniotic fluid volume of 1 L is reached at 36 to 38 weeks gestation. A decrease in volume is usually noted as term approaches, and in the postterm pregnancy clinically apparent oligohydramnios may develop. Oligohydramnios may also occur in association with fetal renal agenesis (Potter syndrome) and in some cases of intrauterine growth retardation.

72. The answer is A. *(Danforth, ed 4. p 331.)* During pregnancy, the plasma volume increases by about 48 percent and the red-cell volume increases by about 30 percent. The rapid increase in the plasma volume occurs during early pregnancy, while the red-cell volume rises more rapidly after the first trimester of pregnancy. As a result, the hematocrit during the first trimester and most of the second trimester of pregnancy could be much lower than normal. The reduction in hematocrit constitutes the "physiological anemia" of pregnancy.

73. The answer is E. *(Pritchard, ed 16. p 3.)* The maternal mortality rate is calculated per 100,000 live births. Although there have been marked advances in prenatal care associated with a declining maternal mortality rate over the past 25 years, there still exist subgroups of the female population at much higher risk. These include black women (apparently because of social and economic conditions), women of high parity, and the older gravida. About 50 percent of maternal deaths in the United States are caused by hemorrhage, hypertension, or infection.

74. The answer is E. *(Pritchard, ed 16. pp 465–466.)* Bloody lochia can persist for up to 2 weeks without indicating an underlying pathology; however, if bleeding continues beyond 2 weeks, it may indicate placental site subinvolution, retention of small placental fragments, or both. At this point, appropriate diagnostic and therapeutic measures should be initiated. The physician should first estimate the blood loss and then perform a pelvic examination in search of uterine subinvolution or tenderness. Excessive bleeding or tenderness should lead the physician to suspect retained placental fragments or endometritis. A larger-than-expected but otherwise asymptomatic uterus supports the diagnosis of subinvolution.

75. The answer is C. *(Pritchard, ed 16. pp 457–458.)* At the time of delivery, the uterus weighs approximately 1000 g. By 1 week postpartum the weight is down to 500 g; by 4 to 6 weeks postpartum it is back to its normal weight, less than 100 g. Most of the weight loss is due to diminution in cell size rather than cell number. Clinically, it is important to keep these facts in mind when examining patients after delivery. If the uterus is still enlarged at the time of the postpartum checkup (usually at 6 weeks), a pathological process, such as subinvolution of the placental site or retained secundines, should be suspected.

76. The answer is A (1, 2, 3). *(Sciarra, ed 2, vol 2, chap 63, pp 1–2.)* Progesterone is thought to result in gradually increasing tidal volume (volume of air moved) to 30 to 40 percent above baseline at term. Although respiratory rate remains unchanged, the increased respiratory minute volume causes a decrease in CO_2 in the alveoli and blood resulting in the "hyperventilation" of the pregnancy.

77. The answer is C (2, 4). *(Burrow, ed 2. pp 36–39.)* During pregnancy fasting blood glucose levels generally decrease, probably because the fetus, needing tremendous amounts of glucose, takes glucose at the expense of the mother. In addition, the maternal response to fasting is accentuated by pregnancy and results in exaggerated starvation ketosis and increased fasting levels of β-hydroxybutyric acid (a ketone body). For a number of reasons, insulin is less effective during pregnancy in diminishing blood glucose. Postprandial blood glucose therefore tends to be higher than in the nonpregnant state, and results of a glucose tolerance test must be interpreted differently. To offset anti-insulin effects, insulin production is augmented during the normal pregnancy, and postprandial insulin levels are increased.

78. The answer is B (1, 3). *(Burrow, ed 2. pp 188–191.)* Probably because of increased estrogen levels, pregnancy is associated with an increase in the amounts of many proteins in the serum, among them thyroxine-binding globulin. In order to maintain normal levels of free thyroxine and triiodothyronine, more total thyroxine must be produced to tie up some of the excess binding sites on the carrier protein. Therefore, the total serum thyroxine concentration increases while the level of free thyroxine stays constant. Thyroid-stimulating hormone (TSH) levels are slightly increased during early pregnancy but by term are back in the normal range, as measured by radioimmunoassay. There are some data to suggest that TSH-like activity also is increased in pregnancy, possibly due to a placental factor, either human chorionic gonadotropin or human chorionic thyrotropin. This explanation applies especially to pregnancies complicated by trophoblastic disease.

79. The answer is C (2, 4). *(Pritchard, ed 16. pp 236–237, 248.)* Plasma fibrinogen levels increase by about 50 percent during pregnancy. This rise is thought to be at least partially responsible for the great increase in the erythrocyte sedimentation rate. The elevated sedimentation rate is consequently almost useless as a significant laboratory value in pregnant women. Serum albumin decreases by about 30 percent during normal pregnancy. Blood urea nitrogen (BUN) decreases markedly during pregnancy; in fact, BUN values falling in the middle of the normal range for nonpregnant women (i.e., around 10 mg/100 ml) may signal significant impairment of renal function in pregnant women.

80. The answer is D (4). *(Burrow, ed 2. pp 40–41.)* The tendency for pregnancy to be diabetogenic is thought to be due mainly to the anti-insulin effects of many of the hormones secreted by the placenta as well as to the possible effect of insulin receptors on the placenta itself. Human chorionic somatomammotropin (also known as human placental lactogen) is present in large amounts in the maternal circulation during the third trimester. Its lipolytic and other actions inhibit glucose uptake and manufacture and therefore stimulate insulin production to rise. Levels of pituitary growth hormone are decreased, especially during late pregnancy, and probably have little to do with increased insulin needs. Estrogen and probably progesterone, both of which are present in increased amounts during pregnancy, probably act as peripheral insulin antagonists and therefore would not lead to decreased insulin secretion.

81. The answer is E (all). *(Burrow, ed 2. p 90.)* Methenamine mandelate (Mandelamine), ampicillin, corticosteroids, and phenolphthalein all can reduce urinary estriol levels. Formaldehyde produced by the acid hydrolysis of methenamine mandelate in the urine can degrade estrogens. Hydrolysis of estrogen conjugates is inhibited by phenolphthalein. Large daily doses of cortisol, which can cross the placenta, suppress fetal adrenal function and therefore inhibit production of estriol precursors. Ampicillin use is thought to cause fecal loss of steroids, which results from an inhibition in the gastrointestinal tract of the hydrolysis of biliary estriol conjugates.

82. The answer is C (2, 4). *(Burrow, ed 2. pp 521–523.)* The diagnosis of breast cancer in pregnancy is more difficult because of the enlargement and hypervascularity of tissue. If associated with lymphatic obstruction, cancer may mimic benign mastitis. Although mammography should not be used for routine screening, it is the diagnostic imaging of choice and can be performed safely with abdominal shielding. All suspicious masses by palpation and either mammography or thermography should have excisional biopsy regardless of pregnancy and definitive surgery, depending on results. Therapeutic abortion is considered only to facilitate treatment of metastatic disease; however, chemotherapy has not been implicated in malformations. Risk of disease recurrence has not been shown to increase with future pregnancies.

83. The answer is E (all). *(Pritchard ed 16. pp 469–470. Speroff, ed 3. p 250.)* Various studies have confirmed all the statements presented in the question. It is thus vital to warn all postpartum women that they can become pregnant even within the first postpartum month whether or not they are breast-feeding.

84. The answer is A (1, 2, 3). *(Speroff, ed 3. pp 246–250.)* The normal sequence of events triggered by suckling is as follows: through a central-nervous-system response, dopamine is decreased in the hypothalamus. Dopamine suppression decreases production of prolactin inhibitory factor (PIF), which normally travels through a portal system to the pituitary gland; because PIF production is decreased, production of prolactin by the pituitary is increased. At this time, the pituitary also releases oxytocin, which causes milk to be expressed from the alveoli into the lactiferous ducts. Suckling suppresses the production of luteinizing-hormone (LH) releasing factor and, as a result, acts as a mild contraceptive (the midcycle LH surge does not occur).

85. The answer is D (4). *(Vandenberg, Clin OB/Gyn 23 (4):1105–1111, 1980.)* Patients at high risk for post partum depression often have previous histories of depression or post partum depression. They are more likely to be primiparous, older or have a long interval between pregnancies, unplanned pregnancies or those with a supportive partner. Prenatal intervention must include the obstetric team with family or peer support when possible. The duration of post partum depression is variable, but occasionally will not resolve without hospitalization, therapy and/or medication.

PRIMARY CARE

History, Physical Examination, and Diagnostic Procedures

DIRECTIONS: Each question below contains five suggested answers. Choose the **one best** response to each question.

86. False positive VDRL tests have been associated with all of the following EXCEPT

(A) narcotic addition
(B) atypical pneumonias
(C) old age
(D) diabetes mellitus
(E) leprosy

87. Routine pelvic examination reveals that a 21-year-old woman has a hooded cervix. This finding is most frequently associated with

(A) pregnancy
(B) traumatic abortion
(C) in utero drug exposure
(D) a prior Shirodkar procedure
(E) a herpesvirus infection

88. The percentage of pregnancy loss that can be attributed to second trimester amniocentesis is approximately

(A) 1 percent
(B) 2 to 3 percent
(C) 3 to 4 percent
(D) 5 percent
(E) more than 5 percent

89. All of the following statements concerning a hysterosalpingogram test for fallopian-tube patency are true EXCEPT that

(A) the contrast medium used may be either oil- or water-soluble
(B) salpingitis isthmica nodosa may be diagnosed with this procedure
(C) abnormalities of the uterine cavity may be diagnosed with this procedure
(D) less than 3 ml of contrast medium should be used to avoid spill from the tubes into the peritoneal cavity
(E) the test may have a therapeutic effect on infertility

90. A 19-year-old nulliparous woman is given a Veneral Disease Research Laboratories (VDRL) test, which is positive at a dilution of 1:4. The diagnositic measure that now should be ordered is a

(A) Wassermann-type test
(B) rapid plasma reagin card test
(C) fluorescent treponemal antibody-absorption (FTA-ABS) test
(D) lumbar puncture and VDRL titer of cerebrospinal fluid
(E) thorough pelvic examination

DIRECTIONS: Each question below contains four suggested answers of which **one or more** is correct. Choose the answer:

A	if	**1, 2, and 3**	are correct
B	if	**1 and 3**	are correct
C	if	**2 and 4**	are correct
D	if	**4**	is correct
E	if	**1, 2, 3, and 4**	are correct

91. A direct Coombs' test is described by which of the following statements?

(1) It can be useful in analyzing the cord blood of babies at risk for Rh disease
(2) It involves an antiglobulin reagent made by immunizing rabbits to human immunoglobulin
(3) It cannot be used to quantify the amount of an antibody present
(4) It can be performed on the sera of pregnant RH-negative women to determine the degree of their Rh sensitization

92. Routine preoperative evaluation of a patient who has a large, fixed, irregular pelvic mass that is highly suggestive of an ovarian tumor should include which of the following diagnostic procedures?

(1) Chest x-ray
(2) Intravenous pyelography
(3) Barium enema
(4) Liver scan

93. A normal gynecological examination in a 65-year-old woman may yield which of the following findings?

(1) A Bartholin's gland that is non-palpable
(2) Atrophy of the labia minora
(3) An ovary that is nonpalpable
(4) Dark menstrual-type blood

94. As a description of a woman's obstetrical history, the digits 7-2-1-6 indicate that she has

(1) given birth to six term infants
(2) had two premature deliveries
(3) been pregnant seven times
(4) had one abortion

95. A young woman develops painful vulvar vesicles, and a herpesvirus hominis type 2 (herpes simplex) infection is suspected. The tests that can be done to confirm this diagnosis include

(1) wet mount with saline
(2) culture for the virus
(3) Gram stain
(4) Papanicolaou (Pap) smear

96. Pelvic examination is an important means of diagnosing ovarian malignancies. An ovarian tumor has an increased likelihood of being malignant if examination reveals that it is

(1) mobile
(2) bilateral
(3) cystic
(4) greater than 10 cm in diameter

SUMMARY OF DIRECTIONS

A	B	C	D	E
1,2,3 only	1,3 only	2,4 only	4 only	All are correct

97. A 23-year-old woman (gravida 2, para 1) wants to know the prenatal diagnosis of her unborn child. Her first child, who was deliverd by cesarean section, had anencephaly. An ultra-sound examination performed 1 week ago (at 15 weeks gestation) revealed an anterior placenta and a fetal biparietal diameter consistent with the gestational age as determined by menstrual history. In advising the woman, the physician should keep which of the following statements in mind?

(1) An elevated level of alpha-fetoprotein in the amniotic fluid may not necessarily indicate a neural tube defect

(2) An elevated level of alpha-fetoprotein in the amniotic fluid is as likely to indicate a closed neural tube defect as an open neural tube defect

(3) The midtrimester ultrasound examination makes the diagnosis of recurrent anencephaly highly unlikely in this instance

(4) Repeated measurement of the concentration of alpha-fetoprotein in maternal serum can substitute for amniocentesis

98. In recording a gynecological history, $15 \times 30 \times 6$ is a very common way to record the menstrual history. The numbers in this formula include reference to which of the following information?

(1) The woman's age

(2) The interval since the woman's last menstrual period in days

(3) The duration of the woman's last menstrual period in days

(4) The woman's age at her first menses

DIRECTIONS: The groups of questions below consist of lettered choices followed by several numbered items. For each numbered item select the **one** lettered choice with which it is **most** closely associated. Each lettered choice may be used once, more than once, or not at all.

Questions 99–105

(A) Turner syndrome
(B) Pituitary adenoma
(C) Asherman syndrome
(D) Testicular feminization
(E) Swyer syndrome
(F) Anorexia nervosa
(G) Sheehan syndrome
(H) Other

99. 1° amenorrhea, infantile female sexual development

100. 1° amenorrhea, short stature, shield chest

101. 1° amenorrhea, normal breast development, absent pubic and axillary hair

102. 2° amenorrhea, postpartum hemorrhage, weight loss, fatigue

103. 2° amenorrhea, postpartum hemorrhage, infertility

104. 2° amenorrhea, weight loss, hyperactivity

105. 2° amenorrhea, galactorrhea

Questions 106–112

For each condition that follows, select the study that would be helpful in detecting that condition in utero.

(A) Fetal chromosome count
(B) Fetal sex determination
(C) Amniotic fluid level of alpha-fetoprotein
(D) Enzyme analysis of cultured amniotic fluid cells
(E) None of the above

106. Meningomyelocele

107. Cystic fibrosis

108. Tay-Sachs disease

109. Klinefelter syndrome

110. Hurler syndrome

111. Translocation Down syndrome

112. Hydrocephaly (without associated spinal cord defects)

Questions 113–115

For each of the descriptions below, select the pelvic type with which it is most likely to be associated.

(A) Anthropoid
(B) Android
(C) Gynecoid
(D) Platypelloid
(E) None of the above

113. Examination of the pelvis reveals prominent ischial spines, a narrow subpubic arch, a narrow high-arched sacrosciatic notch, a straight sacrum, and a shortened posterior sagittal diameter

114. Examination of the pelvis reveals a wide subpubic arch, a curved sacrum, and a shortened anteroposterior diameter

115. Examination of the pelvis reveals a lengthened anteroposterior diameter, a large sacrosciatic notch, prominent ischial spines, and a straight, posteriorly inclined sacrum

History, Physical Examination, and Diagnostic Procedures

Answers

86. The answer is D. *(Parsons, ed 2. p 868.)* The VDRL is a serological test widely used to screen for syphilis. False positives appear in approximately 3 to 4 percent of all VDRL tests performed. If a false positive occurs, a physician first should ensure that the result is not due to technical error and second should consider the various entities that result in false positives at the following rates: leprosy (8 to 28 percent), smallpox vaccination (1 to 2 percent), narcotic addiction (20 to 25 percent), and old age (10 percent of patients between 70 and 80 years of age). Atypical pneumonias have also resulted in false positives. The FTA-ABS treponemal test, which is quite specific, should be used with a borderline or suspected false positive VDRL test.

87. The answer is C. *(Danforth, ed 4. p 895.)* A hooded cervix, a "cockscomb" cervix, and cervical pseudopolyps are common structural changes associated with in utero exposure to diethylstilbestrol or chemically related nonsteroidal estrogens. Cervical erosions are almost always founded in affected individuals, and vaginal adenosis is frequently present. Carcinomas of the vagina are much less frequently diagnosed.

88. The answer is A. *(Thompson, ed 3. p 344.)* A national prospective controlled study, designed to evaluate the safety and accuracy of prenatal genetic diagnosis by early midtrimester amniocentesis, revealed that the incidence of fetal loss in the approximately 1000 women studied did not differ significantly from that of the controls. The incidence of pregnancy loss directly attributable to midtrimester amniocentesis was found to be less than 1 percent. The overall accuracy of midtrimester amniocentesis for prenatal genetic diagnosis was found to be 99.4 percent.

89. The answer is D. *(Speroff, ed 3. pp 475–476.)* A hysterosalpingogram is a procedure in which 3 to 6 ml of either an oil- or water-soluble contrast medium is injected through the cervix in order to outline the uterine cavity and fallopian tubes. Spill of contrast medium into the peritoneal cavity proves patency of the uterine cavity and fallopian tubes. By outlining the cavity, abnormalities such as bicornuate uterus, uterine polyps, submucous myomas, salpingitis isthmica nodosum, and hydrosalpinx can be identified. Some controlled studies have shown a therapeutic effect resulting in an increased rate of pregnancy in infertility patients.

90. The answer is C. *(Wynn, ed 3. pp 184–185.)* Because a positive VDRL test either may indicate the presence of syphilis or may be a biological false positive, a specific treponemal test, such as the fluorescent treponemal antibody-absorption (FTA-ABS) test, is needed to discriminate false positives from true infection. The rapid plasma reagin (RPR) card test and Wassermann-type tests, such as the Kolmer test, are nontreponemal tests and therefore are no more specific than the VDRL test. A lumbar puncture would not be indicated at this point. A pelvic examination may be of little diagnostic use, because chancres often disappear before a VDRL test becomes positive.

91. The answer is A (1, 2, 3). *(Queenan, ed 2. pp 14–15.)* The direct Coombs' test, which uses human antiglobulin derived from immunized rabbits, is performed on blood cells to determine if they are coated with antibody. A direct Coombs' test, therefore, can be useful in analyzing the cord blood of an infant who is at risk for Rh disease. Quantification of antibody titers can be achieved by doing serial dilutions of the indirect Coombs' test, which analyzes serum.

92. The answer is C (1, 2, 3). *(Wynn, ed 3. p 267.)* A chest x-ray, an intravenous pyelogram, and a barium enema all are important in the evaluation of a woman suspected of having an ovarian malignancy. Chest x-rays can reveal occult metastases as well as pleural effusions, which frequently occur in advanced ovarian cancer. Pyelography can assess renal function and reveal ureteral obstruction or deviation as well as duplication of urinary-tract structures. Barium enemas can help distinguish a neoplastic or inflammatory process arising from the colon from extrinsic compression due to an ovarian tumor. A liver scan is not routinely performed, because ovarian cancer usually does not spread hematogenously; a scan is indicated only if liver function tests are abnormal or the liver is palpably enlarged.

93. The answer is A (1, 2, 3). *(Wynn, ed 3. pp 328–330.)* The Bartholin's gland located at the junction of the middle and lower thirds of the vagina is usually not palpable unless it is involved in a cyst or an abscess. The decreased estrogen levels associated with the postmenopausal state are normally associated with atrophic changes of the labia minora, vaginal mucosa, uterus, and ovaries. It is common to be unable to palpate the normal ovary, especially in an obese, uncooperative, or postmenopausal woman. Any bleeding whatsoever in the postmenopausal female should be considered abnormal and should alert the physician to the possibility of a malignancy.

94. The answer is C (2, 4). *Pritchard, ed 16. p 304.)* Describing an obstetrical history by the four-digit system is more comprehensive than merely indicating gravidity and parity. The first digit of the four indicates the number of term infants delivered; the second, the number of premature infants delivered; the third, the number of abortions; and the fourth, the number of children now alive. A woman described as 7-2-1-6, therefore, has had seven term deliveries, two premature deliveries, and one abortion; and six of her children currently are alive.

95. The answer is C (2, 4). *(Danforth, ed 4. p 990.)* Herpesvirus hominis type 2 (herpes simplex) can be cultured readily and rapidly; however, available facilities to perform viral cultures are limited. A Papanicolaou (Pap) smear will show typical herpetic findings (multinucleated giant cells and intranuclear inclusions) in approximately 85 percent of affected women. Wet mounts and Gram stains are inadequate detectors of viral infection.

96. The answer is C (2, 4). *(Wynn, ed 3. p 267.)* Unilateral, cystic, mobile, and small (less than 10 cm) adnexal masses tend to be benign neoplasms. Masses that are bilateral, solid, fixed, and large, on the other hand, more characteristically are malignant and require prompted diagnostic evaluation and treatment. Ascites also is frequently associated with ovarian malignancies.

97. The answer is B (1, 3). *(Pritchard, ed 16. pp 339–344.)* The demonstration by ultrasound examination of a well-defined vertex of normal size can rule out anencephaly. Amniotic fluid levels of alpha-fetoprotein are currently the most reliable tool to detect those neural tube defects not covered by skin (open defects). Elevated levels also may be associated with fetal blood contamination of the amniotic fluid (often due to amniocentesis through an anteriorly implanted placenta) or with a number of fetal disorders. Because maternal serum alpha-fetoprotein levels have been reported to be elevated in only 50 to 70 percent of cases in which the fetus has had an open neural tube defect, its use as the exclusive diagnostic procedure in couples at increased risk for having children with this disorder is not generally recommended.

98. The answer is D (4). *(Wynn, ed 3. pp 5–6.)* The formula $15 \times 30 \times 6$ is a commonly used abbreviation for recording a woman's menstrual history. The first digit refers to the woman's age at the onset of menses (menarche). The second digit refers to the usual interval between menses in days. The third digit refers to the duration of the woman's usual menstrual period in days. Thus, the woman described by this formula was 15 years of age at the onset of menses; her cycle runs approximately 30 days; and each period lasts approximately 6 days.

99–105. The answers are: 99-E, 100-A, 101-D, 102-G, 103-C, 104-F, 105-B.
(Speroff, ed 3. pp 156–164, 173, 177.) After obtaining a history and performing a physical examination, other testing may be helpful in diagnosing causes of amenorrhea. An abnormal karyotype will be seen with Turner syndrome (45,X) testicular feminization (46,XY), and Swyer syndrome (46,XY). Testosterone levels will distinguish between the latter two conditions. Such diagnosis is important because the streak gonads in Swyer syndrome have high potential for transformation and should be removed as soon as diagnosis is made, whereas those in testicular feminization can be retained until after puberty.

Although Asherman syndrome can also occur in the patient with Sheehan syndrome, the latter is typified by pituitary insufficiency rather than end organ dysfunction from scarred endometrial tissue. Anorexia nervosa is dysfunction associated with stress and weight loss, but high cortisol levels are found.

106–112. The answers are: 106-C, 107-E, 108-D, 109-A, 110-D, 111-E, 112-E. *(Burrow, ed 2. pp 118–135.)* Aneuploidy can be detected simply by counting fetal chromosomes; the diagnosis of aneuploid disorders, such as Klinefelter syndrome (47,XXY) and trisomy 21 (classic Down syndrome) can be confirmed by karyotype. Because individuals who have translocation Down syndrome have 46 chromosomes, a chromosome count would be unrewarding; modern chromosome-banding techniques, however, can demonstrate this abnormality during analysis of the karyotype. Although cystic fibrosis is an inherited, autosomal recessive disorder, it cannot be detected prenatally at this time.

Meningomyelocele and other open neural-tube defects have markedly elevated amniotic fluid levels of alpha-fetoprotein, probably as a result of the transudation of this protein across the membrane covering the defect. If a neural-tube defect is completely covered with skin, however, the alpha-fetoprotein level may be within normal limits; an example of such closed defects is hydrocephaly that is not associated with spinal cord lesions.

Tay-Sachs disease results from a defect in the synthesis of hexosaminidase A. Hurler syndrome is caused by a deficiency of the enzyme L-iduronidase. Both disorders can be detected by enzyme analysis of cultured fetal cells grown from amniotic fluid.

113–115. The answers are: 113-B, 114-D, 115-A. *(Pritchard, ed 16. pp 286–288.)* The four general pelvic configurations, named here according to the widely used Caldwell-Moloy classification, may be important indicators of potential problems during labor and delivery. The gynecoid pelvis, the most common type, is generally round, with the transverse diameter being the same as or slightly greater than the anteroposterior diameter.

The anthropoid pelvis is essentially oblong, with the anteroposterior diameter being much greater than the transverse diameter. It is thus a deep, narrow pelvis; characteristically, the ischial spines are prominent and the sacrum is inclined posteriorly.

The android pelvis is often described as triangular. The anterior pelvis is narrowed, with a narrow subpubic angle; but, unlike the anthropoid pelvis, the posterior pelvis is short, with a small posterior sagittal diameter. The spines are prominent in the android pelvis, and the sacrum is straight. Unless it is unusually large, this type of pelvis offers a poor prognosis for delivery.

The rarest pelvic type is the platypelloid ("flat") pelvis. Here the anteroposterior diameter is quite short and the transverse diameter is wide. The subpubic angle is wide and the ischial spines are not prominent. This type of pelvis may cause the vertex to stay in the occiput transverse position until delivery.

Clinical, Behavioral, Medical, and Legal Problems

DIRECTIONS: Each question below contains five suggested answers. Choose the **one best** response to each question.

116. The management of girls who have idiopathic precocious puberty includes

(A) progestin therapy
(B) estrogen therapy
(C) androgen therapy
(D) pelvic irradiation
(E) laparoscopy

117. A 22-year-old woman, gravida 3, para 2 (one abortion), is brought to the hospital because she says she has been raped by a 35-year-old man whom she knows to have had a vasectomy 2 years ago. Both individuals have an A-positive blood type. Which of the following would be most useful to her in the prosecution of this case?

(A) Accurate description of the introitus
(B) Smear for sperm from the cervix
(C) Vaginal washings for acid phosphatase
(D) Specific typing of vaginal washings
(E) Examination of her pubic hair

118. In the experience of Masters and Johnson and other sex therapists, the sexual dysfunction having the lowest cure rate is

(A) premature ejaculation
(B) vaginismus
(C) primary impotence
(D) secondary impotence
(E) female orgasmic dysfunction

119. A 17-year-old girl presents at the emergency room at 6 a.m. with acute urinary retention. On questioning, she states that her menstrual periods have not started, although she does have a monthly attack of mild lower abdominal discomfort, which is relieved by analgesics. Physical examination reveals well-developed secondary sexual characteristics, with an abdominal mass extending up to the level of the umbilicus. A pregnancy test is negative. The most likely diagnosis is

(A) intrauterine fetal death
(B) imperforate hymen
(C) ovarian tumor
(D) tuberculous peritonitis
(E) gestational trophoblastic disease

120. Which of the following statements is true regarding the menarchial female?

(A) Pubic hair growth generally precedes breast budding
(B) Most cycles are anovulatory in the first year of menstruation
(C) Body weight correlates highly on the onset of menarche
(D) the age of menarche bears little association with mother's age of menarche
(E) The mean age of menarche in this country is increasing slightly with each decade

121. The most common cause of precocious puberty in girls is

(A) idiopathic
(B) gonadal tumors
(C) Albright syndrome
(D) hypothyroidism
(E) central nervous system tumors

122. Labial agglutination in a young girl is best treated by

(A) forcible separation
(B) estrogen cream
(C) surgical excision
(D) antibiotics
(E) warm compresses

123. A 46-year-old woman presents with depression, urinary urgency, night sweats, and headaches. On examination she is found to be anovulatory. The most likely diagnosis is

(A) psychosomatic disorder
(B) manic depression
(C) urinary tract infection
(D) tuberculosis with renal involvement
(E) menopause

124. The most frequent cause of a blood discharge from the nipple is

(A) carcinoma of the breast
(B) intraductal papilloma
(C) fibroadenoma
(D) cystosarcoma phyllodes
(E) breast abscess

125. True statements about the creation of the patient-physician relationship include which of the following?

(1) The patient-physician relationship is considered a contract
(2) The patient has the right to accept or reject the physician's proposed service as part of the contract
(3) A consent is not considered valid unless the patient comprehends the involved treatment and its ramifications
(4) If the physician begins treatment, he or she is considered to be involved in the contract.

126. Endocrine-related causes of short stature in young women include

(1) hypothyroidism
(2) adrenal hyperplasia
(3) Cushing's disease
(4) Turner syndrome

DIRECTIONS: Each question below contains four suggested answers of which **one or more** is correct. Choose the answer:

A	if	**1, 2, and 3**	are correct
B	if	**1 and 3**	are correct
C	if	**2 and 4**	are correct
D	if	**4**	is correct
E	if	**1, 2, 3, and 4**	are correct

127. Estrogen administration is considered advantageous in the treatment of perimenopausal women who have

(1) emotional reactions
(2) vasomotor reactions
(3) osteoporosis
(4) epithelial atrophy

128. Delayed puberty should be suspected if

(1) breast budding is still absent by age 13.
(2) 5 years have elapsed between the onset of breast budding and the expected menarche
(3) menarche is delayed beyond 16 years of age
(4) FSH >40 mIU/ml at age 16

129. Primary orgasmic dysfunction in women can be described by which of the following statements?

(1) It can stem from dissatisfaction with a partner's behavior patterns
(2) The influence of orthodox religious beliefs is still of major etiological significance
(3) It can be exacerbated if a partner suffers from premature ejaculation
(4) A woman affected by it has never in her life achieved orgasm

130. A woman may experience orgasm by

(1) clitoral stimulation
(2) vaginal stimulation
(3) dreams
(4) extragenital stimulation

131. Female dyspareunia can be described by which of the following statements?

(1) It rarely affects postmenopausal women
(2) Complaints of pain during penile thrusting usually indicate pelvic pathology
(3) Bacterial vaginal infection is a minor etiological factor
(4) It can develop from sensitivity to intravaginal contraceptive agents

132. Which of the following statements regarding rape by a known versus an unknown assailant are true?

(1) Long-term sexual difficulties arise more frequently when a patient is the victim of rape by an unknown assailant
(2) Rape by a stranger is far more likely to be reported than rape by a known assailant
(3) Sexual adjustment is easier after rape by a known assailant
(4) Many women with sexual dysfunction may in fact be sufferers of "silent rape" syndrome.

133. Dyspareunia may be the result of

(1) psychological etiology
(2) organic causes
(3) birth-control pills with high estrogen content
(4) intrauterine devices

134. Treatment for dysfunctional uterine bleeding may include

(1) progestin therapy
(2) combined birth-control therapy
(3) estrogen therapy
(4) antiprostaglandin therapy

135. The use of estrogen replacement therapy may be hazardous, if not expressly contraindicated, for women who have

(1) impaired hepatic function
(2) thromboembolic disorders
(3) estrogen-dependent tumors
(4) a mother or sister with osteoporosis

136. Although the incidence of rape is increasing in the United States, data indicate that three out of every four rapes still are not reported to law enforcement authorities. True statements about rape include which of the following?

(1) Rape usually results in pregnancy
(2) Many rapes are perpetrated by men who find violence necessary for sexual fulfillment
(3) Tests for venereal disease should not be performed on rape victims immediately following a rape
(4) Rape can cause sexual dysfunction

DIRECTIONS: The groups of questions below consist of lettered choices followed by several numbered items. For each numbered item select the **one** lettered choice with which it is **most** closely associated. Each lettered choice may be used once, more than once, or not at all.

Questions 137–140

The normal stages of breast development are

(A) First
(B) Second
(C) Third
(D) Fourth

137. Pubarche

138. Accelerated growth

139. Menarche

140. Breast development

Questions 141–145

For each of the circumstances of death that might occur in a patient with generalized carcinomatosis, select the correct term used to describe the occurrence.

(A) Natural death
(B) Passive euthanasia
(C) Active euthanasia
(D) Facilitated suicide
(E) Suicide

141. Coincidental myocardial infarction with failure of resuscitative efforts

142. Overdose of barbiturates procured by the patient and administered by the patient without the physician's consent

143. Overdose of barbiturates procured by the physician and administered by the patient with the physician's and patient's consent

144. Overdose of barbiturates procured by the physician and administered by the physician with the physician's and patient's consent

145. Myocardial infarction with no attempt at resuscitative efforts

Clinical, Behavioral, Medical, and Legal Problems

Answers

116. The answer is A. *(Speroff, ed 3. pp. 375–376.)* Progestin therapy is the treatment of choice for girls who have idiopathic precocious puberty. Although progestins cannot cause pubic hair to disappear, they can stop future growth, arrest breast development, and, most important, cause bone growth to decelerate, thus preventing early epiphyseal closure. Estrogen treatment is contraindicated because it can only exacerbate symptoms of precocity and result in short stature. Laparoscopy is not indicated, because most causes of precocious puberty can eventually be determined without surgery.

117. The answer is C. *(American College of Obstetricians and Gynecologists, ACOG Tech Bull 14: July, 1972.)* Although all of the procedures mentioned in the question can be helpful in establishing a case of rape in most situations, the expected lack of sperm and the matching blood types in the situation presented would limit their value in this case. Only the finding of 50 units/ml or more of acid phosphatase in this woman's vagina could be taken as evidence of ejaculation. Her introitus probably would not be injured because of her parity. Foreign pubic hair might only indicate close contact.

118. The answer is C. *(Masters, 1970, p 367.)* In a five-year follow-up study of couples treated by Masters and Johnson, the cure rates for vaginismus and premature ejaculation approached 100 percent. Orgasmic dysfunction was corrected in 80 percent of women, and secondary impotence (impotence despite a history of previous coital success) resolved in 70 percent of men. Primary impotence (chronic and complete inability to maintain an erection sufficient for coitus) was cured only 60 percent of the time. Other therapists report very similar statistics.

119. The answer is B. *(Jeffcoate, ed 4. p 142.)* Patients with imperforate hymen may present to the physician seeking an explanation for amenorrhea; however, in many instances such patients may present as an emergency with abdominal pain with or without an abdominopelvic mass. The intact hymen results in the retention of menstrual blood, which may accumulate over time (often 3 to 4 years). This accumulation of blood in the vagina, uterus, and tubes may result in a pelvic mass that may in turn cause a mechanical obstruction of the urethra. Thus, acute urinary retention with a distended bladder may be the patient's presenting symptoms.

120. The answer is C. *(Romney, ed 2. pp 385–386.)* Although the exact mechanism of menarche is not clearly understood, there is strong evidence to suggest that body weight is the critical variable. There is a high degree of correlation with the growth pattern and the age of menarche of the mother and other female relatives. Menarche occurs approximately 1 to 1 1/2 years after the onset of pubic hair and about 2 years after the appearance of breast buds. Although menses are frequently irregular in the first year or two, studies show that approximately half of the cycles are ovulatory.

121. The answer is A. *(Speroff, ed 3. pp 370–374.)* In North America, any pubertal changes before the age of 8 years in girls and 9 years in boys are regarded as precocious. Although the most common type of precocious puberty in girls is idiopathic, it is essential to ensure close long-term follow-up of these patients to ascertain that there is not serious underlying pathology, such as tumors of the central nervous system or ovary. Only 1 to 2 percent of patients with precocious puberty have an estrogen-producing ovarian tumor as the causative factor. Albright syndrome (polyostotic fibrous dysplasia) is also relatively rare and consists of fibrous dysplasia and cystic degeneration of the long bones, sexual precocity, and café au lait spots on the skin. Hypothyroidism is a cause of precocious puberty in some children, making thyroid function tests mandatory in these cases. Central nervous system tumors as a cause of precocious puberty occur more commonly in boys than in girls.

122. The answer is B. *(Green, ed 3. p 121.)* Labial agglutination is a condition in young girls in which the labia minora are fused together. There is no relationship to either hygiene or presence of vulvovaginitis, and generally speaking the exact reason for the agglutination is unknown. It is important, however, to distinguish this condition from possible congenital anomalies. In asymptomatic patients, no treatment is necessary other than reassurance as this condition will resolve with estrogen production at puberty; however, in patients with symptoms, such as local irritation or difficulty in micturition, separation can be achieved with constant application of estrogen creams. Surgical or forcible separation of the labia should be avoided. Antibiotics and warm compresses are ineffective.

123. The answer is E. *(Speroff, ed 3. pp 114–115.)* The symptoms described in the questions are common symptoms of menopause. They all result primarily from estrogen withdrawal, and most can be reversed by estrogen therapy. "Climacteric" is actually a better word for this complex of symptoms, because the menopause is technically the instant at which menses cease.

124. The answer is B. *(Green, ed 3. pp 616–618.)* Fibroadenomas are the most common benign breast tumors, and they usually do not give rise to any significant symptoms. The diagnosis is often made by the physician on routine examination of the breasts. Intraductal papilloma is the second most common benign breast tumor. Its presenting sign is that of a bloody discharge from the nipple. In order to rule out possible underlying intraductal papillary adenocarcinoma, intraductal papilloma is often treated surgically. Cystosarcoma phyllodes is also a benign tumor that rarely undergoes malignant changes. It can grow to a very large size and surgery is again the recommended treatment. Cancer of the breast can also give rise to a bloody nipple discharge, although not as commonly as intraductal papilloma. A breast abscess may give rise to a purulent nipple discharge.

125. The answer is E (all). *(Kase, p. 929.)* It is extremely difficult to establish if a patient-physician relationship has been created at all. There must be a contract established before responsibility for care can be imposed on the physician. It is considered appropriate for the contract to allow the patient the opportunity to accept or reject treatment proposals.

126. The answer is E (all). *(Speroff, ed 3. p 382.)* Short stature can be associated with adrenal hyperplasia. Cushing's disease, and exogenous cortisone therapy. These factors cause short stature by increasing cortisol levels and, as a result, stimulating epiphyseal closure. Individuals who have Turner syndrome also are characterized by short stature, due to a lack of estrogen production. Hypothyroidism and hypopituitarism can cause short stature in affected girls.

127. The answer is E (all). *(Speroff, ed 3. pp 116–123.)* There is good evidence that estrogen reduces anxiety, depression, and other emotional reactions that can accompany menopause. Estrogens also are helpful in retarding osteoporosis, although their use cannot replace the calcium that already has been lost. The clearest response to estrogen therapy is by the autonomic nervous system; relief from vasomotor reactions, such as hot flashes, by the use of estrogens is significant. A variety of other disturbing symptoms related to epithelial atrophy, such as dyspareunia and urinary urgency, may also be reversed with estrogen therapy.

128. The answer is E (all). *(Kase, p 247.)* Significant emotional concerns develop when puberty is delayed. By definition, if breast development has not begun by age 13, delayed puberty should be suspected. Menarche usually follows 6 months to 1 year after breast development, and if menarche is delayed beyond age 16 delayed puberty should be investigated. Appropriate laboratory tests should be ordered. An FSH >40mIU/ml suggests hypergonadotropic hypergonadism as a cause of delayed maturation.

129. The answer is E (all). *(Masters, 1970, pp 227–237.)* Many factors can contribute to the development of primary orgasmic dysfunction in women. By definition, these women will not have been able to achieve orgasm through any physical means at any time in their lives; reasons for their dysfunction can include the influence of orthodox religious beliefs, dissatisfaction with their partners' behavioral or social traits, past trauma (such as rape), or rigid familial sexual proscriptions. Sexual dysfunction, particularly premature ejaculation in a male partner, can reinforce a woman's orgasmic dysfunction.

130. The answer is E (all). *(Kase, p. 972.)* Sexual ability depends on education, experimentation, and past experience. Sexual orgasm may occur through a variety of routes: direct stimulation of the clitoris, vaginal stimulation, dreams, or stimulation of extragenital erogenous zones. There is no physiologic difference in these orgasms.

131. The answer is D (4). *(Masters, 1970, pp 266–288.)* Aside from psychological causes, female dyspareunia also can stem from a number of physical disorders. Infection of the vaginal barrel, such as with *Escherichia coli* or *Streptococcus faecalis,* can cause distressful burning and aching during and after coition. Insufficient vaginal lubrication also can cause dyspareunia; this condition can occur in postmenopausal women who are not receiving estrogen replacement therapy. Sensitivity to intravaginal chemical contraceptives and irritation of the clitoris, vaginal outlet, or labia can lead to dyspareunia. A woman's complaint of pain during penile thrusting is difficult to evaluate; although this pain can indicate pelvic disorders, such as laceration of uterine ligaments, it also frequently stems from a desire to avoid intercourse.

132. The answer is C (2, 4). *(Kase, p. 989)* Psychological trauma is far greater when the victim knows the rapist. The victim is less likely to report a rape when she knows the assailant and sexual dysfunction is more difficult to resolve. A woman complaining of sexual dysfunction should be carefully but gently questioned about the use of sexual force in the past.

133. The answer is E (all). *(Kase, p. 975.)* Guilt or fear are known to inhibit arousal capability. There are numerous organic reasons for dyspareunia involving the vagina, uterus, ovary, or external genitalia. High estrogen pills may alter vaginal pH, leading to vaginal dryness and painful intercourse. The IUD may cause irritability that is exacerbated by intercourse.

134. The answer is E (all). *(Kase, pp 265–266.)* Dysfunctional uterine bleeding is usually a result of anovulation. Progesterone therapy followed by withdrawal will cause a sloughing of the unstable endometrium. A short-term, large-dose, combined birth-control therapy will frequently rehabilitate the bleeding endometrium. After the withdrawal bleed, the patient can be started on a low-dose cyclic combination of birth-control pills to regulate the menstrual flow. Estrogen therapy is useful on a short-term basis when the bleeding is from inadequate estrogen stimulation of endometrium. Prostaglandin synthetase inhibitors have been shown to decrease menstrual blood loss.

135. The answer is A (1, 2, 3). *(Speroff, ed 3. p 124.)* The use of estrogen replacement therapy can be deleterious for women who have thromboembolic symptoms. Because the liver is influenced significantly by estrogens, which can affect the function of hepatic cell enzymes and production of lipids and lipoproteins, the effects of hepatic impairment can be exacerbated by estrogen therapy. The existence of estrogen-dependent tumors is a contraindication to estrogen use. The long-term disabilities of osteoporosis may be ameliorated with estrogen therapy.

136. The answer is C (2, 4). *(American Medical Association Committee on Human Sexuality, pp 138–139.)* Although rape does not usually cause pregnancy, it can result in numerous emotional and physical sequelae, including sexual dysfunction, venereal disease, hatred and fear of men, and feelings of guilt. A physician's responsibility to a rape victim is to make sure she is protected prophylactically against pregnancy, to carefully record medical evidence of the rape, and to provide counseling. Although tests for venereal disease immediately following a rape could not yet be positive as a result of the rape and although the testing itself can be emotionally harmful, for medicolegal reasons these tests should be performed immediately to document absence of disease in the victim at the time of the rape. In one study of sexual offenders, the most common type of offender was a man who randomly selected unknown victims and found violence to be necessary for sexual fulfillment.

137–140. The answers are: 137-C, 138-A, 139-D, 140-B. *(Kase, p 246.)* The first sign of puberty is usually the accelerated growth spurt followed by breast budding. Usually pubic hair will follow breast buds by a couple of months. Menarche is the culmination of puberty.

141–145. The answers are: 141-A, 142-E, 143-D, 144-C, 145-B. *(Romney, ed 2. pp 49–52.)* With increasing frequency physicians are called upon to become involved in the bioethical considerations of the circumstances surrounding death. The physician should be familiar with the terms used in order to better understand the debates on the moral philosophical issues of this matter. Negative or passive euthanasia is the deliberate withholding or nonadministration of an agent without which the occurrence of death and perhaps its time of occurrence are reasonably foreseeable, whether it is preventable or not. Positive or active euthanasia is described as an act in which a person, other than the person dying, administers an agent that induces an intentional "good" death. Facilitated suicide is the induction of one's own death after someone else has purposefully made available the agent of death. The dying person may then exercise choice to use or not use the means of death made easily available to her or him. Suicide is the induction of one's own death by the administration of a lethal agent not intentionally procured by someone else.

Contraception, Abortion, and Sterilization

DIRECTIONS: Each question below contains five suggested answers. Choose the **one best** response to each question.

146. Which of the following statements is the best explanation for the mechanism of the action of the IUD?

(A) Hyperperistalsis of the fallopian tubes accelerates the transport of the ovum, thereby preventing fertilization
(B) The IUD causes a bacterial endometritis that interferes in implantation
(C) The IUD produces menorrhagia, and the embryo is aborted in the heavy menstrual flow
(D) A sterile inflammatory reaction of the endometrium to the IUD prevents implantation
(E) A hormonal imbalance is caused by the IUD.

147. The major cause of oral-contraceptive failure resulting in an unplanned pregancy is

(A) breakthrough ovulation at midcycle
(B) frequency of intercourse
(C) incorrect use of oral-contraceptives
(D) gastrointestinal malabsorption
(E) development of antibodies

148. A pregnancy of approximately 10 weeks gestation is confirmed in a 30-year-old woman (gravida 5, para 4) with an intrauterine device (IUD) in place. The patient expresses a strong desire for the pregnancy to be continued. On examination the strings of the IUD are protruding from the cervical os. The most appropriate course of action would be

(A) leave the IUD in place without any other treatment
(B) leave the IUD in place and continue prophylactic antibiotics throughout pregnancy
(C) remove the IUD immediately
(D) terminate the pregnancy because of the near certain risk of infection, abortion, or both
(E) perform laparoscopy to rule out an ectopic pregnancy

149. Birth-control pills have been associated with hepatic adenomas. Most of these tumors are

(A) benign
(B) hormone producing
(C) diabetogenic
(D) associated with thromboembolism
(E) associated with urinary tract infections

150. Techniques for second trimester abortions include all of the following EXCEPT

(A) dilitation and evacuation
(B) prostaglandin E_2 vaginal suppositories
(C) intraamniotic oxytocin
(D) intraamniotic prostaglandin $F_2 \alpha$
(E) intraamniotic hypertonic saline

151. The manufacture of ethinyl estradiol was an important breakthrough in the development of oral contraceptives, because the agent was discovered to be

(A) an especially effective estrogen
(B) orally active
(C) less potent and therefore better tolerated than diethylstilbestrol
(D) the endogenously active form of estrogen
(E) an estrogen with a unique action on the hypothalamus

DIRECTIONS: Each question below contains four suggested answers of which **one or more** is correct. Choose the answer:

A	if	**1, 2, and 3**	are correct
B	if	**1 and 3**	are correct
C	if	**2 and 4**	are correct
D	if	**4**	is correct
E	if	**1, 2, 3, and 4**	are correct

152. Which of the following is/are effective for postcoital contraception?

(1) Diethylstilbestrol, 25 mg bid for 5 days
(2) Conjugated estrogens, 30 mg for 5 days
(3) Ethinyl estradiol, 5 mg per day for 5 days
(4) Ovral 2 tabs, PO q2h for 1 day

153. Coitus interruptus (withdrawal) often fails as a method of birth control, because

(1) prostatic secretions containing sperm are released during the excitement and plateau phases of sex response
(2) pelvic thrusting becomes involuntary before ejaculation occurs
(3) many men start ejaculating before they realize it
(4) Cowper's gland secretions often contain sperm

154. Midtrimester intentional abortion by instillation of hypertonic saline into the amniotic cavity may be

(1) regulated by state law
(2) followed by Rh sensitization
(3) followed by disseminated intravascular coagulation
(4) followed by permanent hypertension

155. In patients taking combination-type birth-control pills, altered metabolic functions may include

(1) a decrease in glucose tolerance
(2) an increase in binding globulins
(3) an increase in sodium sulfobromophthalein (Bromsulphalein) retention
(4) an increase in triglycerides

156. The theoretical effectiveness of a given contraceptive is affected by

(1) patient motivation
(2) its relationship to the act of coitus
(3) its ease of use
(4) its antifertility action

157. A woman who is 12 weeks pregnant undergoes an outpatient suction abortion. She returns three days later with a temperature of 39.2°C (102.5°F), lower abdominal cramps, and vaginal bleeding. The uterus is boggy on examination. Appropriate therapy should include

(1) culture and Gram stain of the endocervix
(2) culture of venous blood
(3) antibiotic therapy
(4) uterine curettage

SUMMARY OF DIRECTIONS

A	B	C	D	E
1,2,3 only	1,3 only	2,4 only	4 only	All are correct

158. True statements regarding operative procedures for sterilization include which of the following?

(1) They can be performed immediately postpartum
(2) They have become the most common method of contraception for white couples between 20 and 40 years of age in the United States
(3) They can be considered effective immediately in females (bilateral tubal ligation)
(4) They can be considered effective immediately in males (vasectomy)

159. Progestational agents in birth-control pills have which of the following actions?

(1) Inhibition of secretion of luteinizing hormone
(2) Endometrial decidualization
(3) Thickening of cervical mucus
(4) Prevention of irregular menses

160. The insertion of an IUD would be contraindicated in a 24-year-old woman under which of the following conditions?

(1) A recent, unexplained, abnormal Papanicolaou (Pap) smear
(2) Nulligravid with multiple partners
(3) Previously treated epsiodes of pelvic inflammatory disease
(4) The presence of menses

161. A 26-year-old woman, who comes to your office to renew her supply of birth-control pills, has mild hypertension, truncal obesity, and acne. Laboratory evaluation reveals that her serum levels of free cortisol are increased; this increase could be due to which of the following reasons?

(1) Cushing disease
(2) Displacement of cortisol from transocrotin by progesterone
(3) Estrogen-related interference of the liver's ability to metabolize cortisol
(4) An increase in ACTH production caused by ingestion of birth-control pills

DIRECTIONS: The groups of questions below consist of lettered choices followed by several numbered items. For each numbered item select the **one** lettered choice with which it is **most** closely associated. Each lettered choice may be used once, more than once, or not at all.

Questions 162–165

For each method of surgical sterilization described below select the name of the procedure.

(A) Irving technique
(B) Pomeroy method
(C) Uchida method
(D) Fimbriectomy

162. The distal segment of the fallopian tube is removed either vaginally or abdominally

163. A plain catgut ligature is placed around a knuckle of tube, which is then excised

164. The serosa of the tube is stripped from the muscular portion and 5 cm of tube is excised. The stump is ligated and the edges of the serosa are tied around the distal tube

165. The tube is transected in the midportion and the proximal stump is buried into the myometrium

Questions 166–170

For each description that follows, select the type of abortion with which it is most commonly associated.

(A) Spontaneous abortion
(B) Threatened abortion
(C) Habitual abortion
(D) Missed abortion
(E) Medical therapeutic abortion

166. Occurs in 20 percent of all pregnancies

167. Occurs in 10 percent of all pregnancies

168. Blighted ovum is responsible for 50 percent

169. May be associated with coagulation defect

170. Not possible with the first pregnancy

Questions 171–177

For the following methods of contraception select the most appropriate use effectiveness rate.

(A) 80
(B) 40
(C) 15 to 25
(D) 3 to 10
(E) 5 to 25

171. Rhythm

172. IUD

173. Diaphragm

174. Postcoital douche

175. Oral contraceptive

176. Condom and spermicidal agent

177. Condom alone

Questions 178–182

For each description that follows, select the pharmacological agent with which it is most likely to be associated.

(A) Testosterone
(B) Mestranol
(C) Norethindrone
(D) Clomiphene
(E) Medroxyprogesterone acetate

178. A progestin commonly used in oral contraceptives

179. An orally active estrogen

180. Commercially marketed as Depo-Provera

181. Nonsteroidal very weak estrogen

182. An agent that causes an increase in endogenous estrogen

Questions 183–188

For each situation listed below, select the most appropriate response.

(A) Stop pills and resume after 7 days
(B) Continue pills as usual
(C) Continue pills and use an additional form of contraception
(D) Take an additional pill
(E) Stop pills and seek a medical examination

183. Nausea during first cycle of pills

184. No menses during 7 days following 21-day cycle of correct use

185. Forgot pill 1 day

186. Forgot pill 10 continuous days

187. Light bleeding at midcycle during first month on pill

188. Hemoptysis

Contraception, Abortion, and Sterilization

Answers

146. The answer is D. *(Kase, p 1038.)* It is currently believed that alternation in the cellular and biochemical components of the endometrium occur with the IUD and an inflammatory reaction results after insertion. Polymorphonuclear leukocytes, giant cells, plasma cells, and macrophages are seen in the endometrium after exposure to all IUDs. Biochemical changes in the endometrium include changing levels of lysosomal hydrolases, glycogen deposition, oxygen composition, total proteins, acid and alkaline phosphatases, urea phospholipids, and RNA/DNA ratios. IUDs treated with copper and progesterone exert additional effects.

147. The answer is C. *(Kase, p 1010.)* The pregnancy rate with birth-control pills, based on theoretical effectiveness, is 0.1 percent. However, the pregnancy rate in actual use is 0.7 percent. This increase is due to incorrect use of the pills. Breakthrough ovulation on combination birth-control pills is thought to be a very rare occurrence. The effectiveness of the pills is not related to sexual frequency, gastrointestinal disturbances, or the development of antibodies.

148. The answer is C. *(Kase, pp 1051–1052)* Although there is an increased risk of spontaneous abortion, and a small risk of infection, an intrauterine pregnancy can occur and continue successfully to term with an intratuerine device (IUD) in place. However, if the patient wishes to keep the pregnancy and if the strings are visible, the IUD should be removed in an attempt to reduce the risk of infection, abortion, or both. Although the percentage of ectopic pregnancies may be increased, the majority of pregnancies occurring with an IUD are intrauterine. Therefore, in the absence of signs and symptoms suggestive of a ectopic pregnancy, laparoscopy is not indicated.

149. The answer is A. *(Kase, pp 1022–1023.)* Focal nodular hyperplasia of the liver and hepatic adenomas are unusual complications of birth-control pills. Even though most pill-induced hepatic adenomas are benign, they have been associated with rupture and serious hemorrhage. Birth-control pills on occasion may be associated with such diverse complications as urinary tract infection, thromboembolism, altered carbohydrate metabolism, and hormonal effects. These changes are ascribed to the pills and are not signs of a hepatic tumor.

150. The answer is C. *(Pritchard, ed 16. p 603.)* All the methods listed are used for second trimester terminations except intraamniotic oxytocin. Induction of labor with oxytocin in the second trimester requires very large doses; however, oxytocin can be used intravenously to augment contractions once labor has been initiated.

151. The answer is B. *(Speroff, ed 3. pp 410–411.)* An ethinyl group added at the 17 position makes ethinyl estradiol a very potent, orally active estrogen. Until this discovery in 1938, no orally effective estrogen had been manufactured. The effects of ethinyl estradiol on the hypothalamus and peripheral receptors are not different from other estrogens. Its contraceptive properties are therefore similar to other estrogens. The contraceptive properties of ethinyl estradiol are not significantly different from other estrogens. Ethinyl estradiol is up to 25 times as potent as diethylstilbestrol.

152. The answer is E (all). *(Speroff, ed 3. p 442.)* Estrogen in large doses is effective as a "morning after" contraceptive. The mechanism of action is unclear. Antiemetic agents are usually prescribed to ease the nausea frequently seen as a side effect.

153. The answer is C (2, 4). *(Masters, 1966. pp 293, 298.)* Cowper's gland secretions, released in late plateau phase, are thought to contain sperm. Prostatic secretions probably do not contribute to this preejaculatory emission. At the very end of the plateau phase, voluntary pelvic thrusting can become involuntary, therefore making withdrawal of the penis difficult. For 2 or 3 seconds before ejaculation, prostatic secretions fill the prostatic urethra, resulting in a feeling that the ejaculation is coming ("ejaculatory inevitability").

154. The answer is A (1, 2, 3). *(Kase, p 1063.)* Saline abortions performed in the midtrimester may be followed by significant fetomaternal transfusion. Rh_o immunoglobulin (RhoGAM) should therefore be administered to Rh-negative patients under the same conditions as with a full-term pregnancy. Although state law may not prohibit midtrimester abortions, it may regulate their performance to protect maternal health. Although they are infrequent, many serious complications may follow a saline abortion. Among these are encephalopathy, hypernatremia, hemoglobinuria, cardiac arrest, tissue necrosis, and disseminated intravascular coagulation. Although acute cardiovascular reactions, including hypertension, do occur, they are not permanent.

155. The answer is E (all.) *(Kase, pp 1018–1020.)* Combination-type oral contraceptives are potent systemic steroids that may cause many detectable alterations in metabolic function, such as increases in binding globulins, Bromsulphalein re-

tention, triglycerides, and total phospholipids, and a decrease in glucose tolerance. Thus, the benefits of birth-control pills must be weighed carefully against
the added risks in patients with diabetes, cardiovascular disease, or liver disease.

156. The answer is D (4.) *(Kase, p 1010.)* The theoretical effectiveness is the
antifertility effectiveness of the contraceptive observed under optimal conditions,
that is, when used properly and regularly. Use effectiveness, on the other hand,
describes the actual effectiveness observed under realistic conditions. Use effectiveness is therefore influenced by such factors as cost, convenience of use, relationship to coitus, and the requirement for repeated patient motivation.

157. The answer is E (all.) *(Monif, pp 278–280.)* Culture and Gram stain of the
endocervix are important in directing antibiotic therapy of women who have had
septic abortions. Blood cultures also can be very helpful, because they are positive
in 30 to 50 percent of patients who have an abortion-related infection. Broad-
spectrum antibiotic therapy is, of course, indicated. Moreover, in a woman who
has a fever, cramps, and vaginal bleeding following an abortion, retention of conception products must be suspected, and curettage should be performed.

158. The answer is A (1, 2, 3). *(Kase, pp 1067–1070.)* Sterilization has become
the most commonly utilized method of contraception in the United States for white
couples between 20 and 40 years of age. In an otherwise uncomplicated pregnancy, a tubal ligation can, if desired, be performed in the immediate postpartum
period. Unless the woman has already conceived at the time of the procedure, the
contraceptive effect is immediate. Vasectomy in the male, however, should not be
considered effective until an examination of the ejaculate is sperm-free on two
successive occasions.

159. The answer is A (1, 2, 3). *(Speroff, ed 3. pp 414–417.)* Progestational
agents in oral contraceptives work by a negative-feedback mechanism to inhibit
the secretion of luteinizing hormone and, as a result, prevent ovulation. They also
cause decidualization and atrophy of the endometrium, hence making implantation impossible. In addition, cervical mucus, which at ovulation is thin and watery,
is changed by the influence of progestational agents to a tenacious compound that
severely limits sperm motility; and some evidence indicates that they may change
ovum and sperm migration patterns within the reproductive system. Progestins
do not prevent irregular bleeding. Estrogen in birth-control pills enhances the negative feedback of the progestins and stabilizes the endometrium to prevent irregular menses.

160. The answer is A (1, 2, 3) *(Kase, pp 1046–1047.)* Insertion of an IUD in the face of an unexplained abnormal Pap smear may interfere with diagnosis and also conceivably disseminate abnormal cells. Bacterial contamination associated with insertion into a patient whose local host defenses are impaired by tissues damaged from previous pelvic inflammatory disease could result in acute reinfection. In nulligravid patients, the risk of sterility resulting from complications of an IUD does not absolutely contraindicate its use; however, such risk should be explained in detail to the patient in order that other equally effective methods of contraception can be explored. The risk of pelvic inflammatory disease increases with the number of partners. Insertion of an IUD during menses eases the insertion and also gives added assurance against placement into a pregnant uterus.

161. The answer is A (1, 2, 3). *(Speroff, ed 3. p 426.)* The clinical symptoms and increased free cortisol levels of the woman described in the question suggest Cushing's disease. Her elevated cortisol levels also could be due to certain metabolical effects of birth-control pills. It was once believed that the pill increased the transcortin level but not the free cortisol level; however, the free cortisol level may in fact increase because of displacement of free cortisol from transcortin by progesterone. The high levels of estrogen in women taking birth-control pills can hinder the liver's ability to metabolize cortisol, resulting in higher-than-normal cortisol levels. If the pill has any effect on pituitary production of ACTH, it is a suppressive one.

162–165. The answers are: 162-D, 163-B, 164-C, 165-A. *(Kase, pp 1067–1069.)* There are many surgical methods for female sterilization. Minilaparotomy and postpartum abdominal, vaginal, and laparoscopic approaches are all effective means to prevent pregnancies. Of the abdominal routes, the Pomeroy method is the most commonly used because of its simplicity and effectiveness.

166–170. The answers are: 166-B, 167-A, 168-A, 169-D, 170-C. *(Pritchard, ed 16. pp 588–597.)* Abortion is defined as a pregnancy that terminates before the fetus is suffiently developed to survive. Many different types of abortion have been identified.

Threatened abortion signified by vaginal bleeding in early pregnancy occurs in about 20 percent of all pregnancies; in about 50 percent of these, the cause is implantation of a normal ovum. In these cases of implantation bleeding, the bleeding would be expected to cease and the pregnancy to continue in a normal fashion. In the other 50 percent of threatened abortions (10 percent of all pregnancies) the bleeding will continue and spontaneous abortion will follow. A blighted ovum is the most common cause (50 percent) for spontaneous abortion.

Occasionally the products of conception will die, yet spontaneous abortion does not ensue. This prolonged retention of a dead fetus in the first half of pregnancy is termed a missed abortion. On rare occasions this prolonged retention of dead tissue can be associated with disseminated intravascular coagulation, a serious coagulation disorder.

Habitual abortion is generally considered to be three or more consecutive spontaneous abortions. Although there are many causes for this disorder, it is probably a chance phenomenon most of the time.

171–177. The answers are: 171-B, 172-D, 173-C, 174-A, 175-E, 176-E, 177-C. *(Kase, p 1011).* There are two methods of describing the effectiveness of contraceptive agents. The theoretical or method effectiveness rate and the actual use effectiveness rate. When comparing different methods it is important to use comparable figures.

The effectiveness of the rhythm method is influenced by the woman's ability to predict the time of ovulation from the regularity of her menses. It is also influenced by the woman's motivation to successfully abstain from intercourse during the 10 days around suspected ovulation. The menstrual and ovulatory irregularities and lapses in the woman's motivation account for a pregnancy rate of 40 with the rhythm method.

In contrast to the rhythm method, the IUD requires little or no action on the part of the woman. For this reason the device's actual use effectiveness approaches its maximal theoretical effectivness with a pregnancy rate of 3–10. Unrecognized expulsion or misplaced insertion of the IUD are responsible for most failures.

The vaginal diaphragm and the condom are barrier contraceptives in that for each act of sexual intercourse they pose a barrier between the sperm ejaculate and the endocervical canal. In theory, both can be very effective. However, both require recurrent motivation for application with each act of intercourse. Lapses in motivation are not uncommon, and there is a pregnancy rate of 15–25 for each of these two methods. The condom used with a spermicidal agent is very effective, more than either used alone.

The pregnancy rate with postcoital douching is almost the same as that for unprotected intercourse (80). This lack of effectiveness is readily explained by the extremely rapid progression of motile sperm into the endocervical canal, coupled with the failure of a vaginal douche to reach this area.

Combined oral contraceptive birth-control pills are clearly the most effective reversible contraceptive currently available. With correct use many studies report a contraceptive effectiveness that approaches 100 percent (pregnancy rate less than 0.1). This extreme effectiveness is best explained by the pills multiplicity of actions i.e., suppression of ovulation, hostility of cervical mucus to sperm penetration, and hostility of atrophic endometrium to the implantation of a conceptus. Failure to take the pills with punctilious regularity is responsible for most failures.

178–182. The answers are: 178-C, 179-C, 180-E, 181-D, 182-D. *(Speroff, ed 3. pp 410–415, 439–440, 524–525.)* Ethinyl estradiol and mestranol are the two active synthetic estrogens used in birth-control pills (mestranol is employed more commonly than ethinyl estradiol). An ethinyl group at the 17 position makes these estrogens orally active.

By removing the 19 carbon from testosterone, a nontestosterone, orally active progestational agent (a 19-nortestosterone) is obtained. Norethindrone is the most commonly used progestational agent of this type in birth-control pills.

The progestational agent medroxyprogesterone acetate (Depo-Provera), along with chlormadinone, has been noted to produce benign breast tumors in beagle puppies; when estrogens were administered at the same time, however, this effect could not be reproduced.

Clomiphene is a nonsteroidal very weak estrogenic agent. By inhibiting hypothalamic regulation of estrogen production, causing estrogen levels to increase, clomiphene can promote ovulation in certain groups of anovulatory women.

183–188. The answers are: 183-B, 184-B, 185-D, 186-C, 187-B, 188-E. *(Speroff, ed 3. pp 417–418, 431, 435–436.)* Common side effects of birth-control pills include nausea, breakthrough bleeding, bloating, and leg cramps. If these side effects are experienced in the first two or three cycles of pills, when they are most common, the pills may be safely continued as these effects usually remit spontaneously.

On occasion, following correct use of a full cycle of pills, withdrawal bleeding may fail to occur (silent menses). Pregnancy is a very unlikely explanation for this event; therefore, pills should be resumed as usual (after 7 days) just as if bleeding had occurred. However, if a second consecutive period has been missed, pregnancy should be more seriously considered and ruled out by a pregnancy test, medical examination, or both.

Women occasionally forget to take pills; however, when only a single pill has been omitted, it can be taken immediately in addition to the usual pill at the usual time. This single-pill omission is associated with little if any loss in effectiveness. If three or more pills are omitted, the pill should be resumed as usual, but an additional contraceptive method (e.g., condoms) should be used through one full cycle.

Although most side effects caused by birth-control pills can be considered minor, serious side effects do sometimes occur. A painful swollen calf may signal thrombophlebitis. Hemoptysis may signal pulmonary embolism. Either of these circumstances should be considered a medical emergency, and immediate medical attention should be sought.

NORMAL
PREGNANCY

The Fetus, Placenta, and Newborn

DIRECTIONS: Each question below contains five suggested answers. Choose the **one best** response to each question.

189. Congenital heart malformations occur with exposure to teratogenic agents at what postmenstrual age?

(A) 2 to 3 weeks
(B) 4 to 5 weeks
(C) 6 to 8 weeks
(D) 9 to 12 weeks
(E) None of the above

190. The normal umbilical cord contains which of the following systems of blood vessels?

(A) One artery and one vein
(B) One artery and two veins
(C) Two arteries and one vein
(D) Two arteries and two veins
(E) None of the above

191. Epidemiologic or clinical studies support all of the following statements concerning the effects of cigarette smoking during pregnancy EXCEPT that

(A) there is a reduction in birth weight of the offspring of smokers when compared to matched controls
(B) the incidence of premature labor is not statistically significant in women who smoke
(C) the incidence of pregnancy-induced hypertension is increased in women who smoke
(D) the effects of smoking are directly proportional to the number of cigarettes smoked
(E) the number of cigarettes smoked daily after the third month of gestation is more important than the number smoked before that time

192. The pH of a fetal scalp sample is abnormal if it is less than

(A) 7.25
(B) 7.30
(C) 7.35
(D) 7.40
(E) 7.45

193. A syndrome of multiple congenital anomalies, including microcephaly, cardiac anomalies, and growth retardation, has been described in children of women who are heavy users of

(A) amphetamines
(B) barbiturates
(C) heroin
(D) methadone
(E) ethyl alcohol

194. During labor, deceleration of the fetal heart rate correlates most closely with which of the following fetal values?

(A) Arterial pH
(B) Arterial P_{O_2}
(C) Arterial P_{CO_2}
(D) Central venous pressure
(E) Venous potassium levels

195. One or more accessory lobes of placenta with vascular connection occur in

(A) succinturate placenta
(B) circumvallate placenta
(C) fenistrate placenta
(D) marginate placenta
(E) all of the above

196. At 20 weeks gestation, the crown-rump length of the fetus is approximately

(A) 9 cm
(B) 12 cm
(C) 14 cm
(D) 16 cm
(E) 19 cm

DIRECTIONS: Each question below contains four suggested answers of which **one or more** is correct. Choose the answer:

A	if	**1, 2, and 3**	are correct
B	if	**1 and 3**	are correct
C	if	**2 and 4**	are correct
D	if	**4**	is correct
E	if	**1, 2, 3, and 4**	are correct

197. A woman at 16 weeks gestation presents for a routine exam, and an ulcerative 0.5-cm lesion is observed lateral to her right labium. She reports that she has had similar irritations there for 3 years. As appropriate management steps you should

(1) verify diagnosis by culture of the lesion
(2) recommend delivery by cesarean section if lesion has healed and membranes rupture 8 hours before arrival at hospital
(3) recommend delivery by cesarean section if cervical lesions or positive cervical cultures are noted in last 4 weeks of gestation and membranes are intact
(4) recommend abortion if culture is positive because of high frequency of transplacental congenital infection in early pregnancy

198. True statements about monozygotic twinning include which of the following?

(1) It tends to run in families
(2) It frequently is associated with pregnancies induced by clomiphene citrate
(3) It is more common that dizygotic twinning
(4) It occurs in approximately 1 pregnancy in 250

199. Substances that are normally found in higher concentrations in the maternal blood than in fetal or umbilical cord blood include

(1) immunoglobulin G (IgG)
(2) immunoglobulin M (IgM)
(3) gamma chains of hemoglobin
(4) fibrinogen

200. Signs of fetal postmaturity that may be noted prior to delivery include

(1) oligohydramnios
(2) maternal edema
(3) meconium-stained amniotic fluid
(4) maternal weight loss

201. Information about which of the following can be obtained by ultrasonography in the third trimester?

(1) Anencephaly and major neural tube defects
(2) Fetal death
(3) Polyhydramnios
(4) Most accurate dating of gestational age

202. True statements about the lecithin-to-sphingomyelin ratio include which of the following?

(1) It can reflect total muscle mass of the fetus
(2) It rises later than normal if toxemia of pregnancy has developed
(3) It rises earlier than normal if erythroblastosis fetalis has developed
(4) It can reflect fetal surfactant production

203. Congenital anomolies have been described in humans for all of the following anticonvulsants EXCEPT

(1) diphenylhydantoin
(2) valproic acid
(3) trimethadione
(4) carbamazepine

204. A full-term infant is found to have a heart rate less than 100 beats per minute at 1 minute after birth. The infant does not cry and has central cyanosis, slow and irregular respiration, and some flexion of the extremities. The obstetrician should

(1) start immediate resuscitation
(2) give the infant a 1-minute Apgar score of 3
(3) call for pediatric consultation
(4) assume that adequate ventilation will correct the respiratory depression

205. Acute obstruction of the umbilical circulation has been found experimentally to provoke which of the following responses?

(1) A rapid fall in fetal central venous pressure
(2) An almost immedite fall in fetal heart rate
(3) A rapidly mediated humoral effect on the fetal heart
(4) A rapidly mediated response by the fetal heart that can be affected by cutting the vagi

206. Severe fetal or neonatal infection can result from maternal infection near term by which of the following viruses?

(1) Group B coxsackievirus
(2) Rubella virus
(3) Chickenpox virus
(4) Herpesvirus hominis, type 2

207. Maternal diabetes mellitus is associated with which of the following symptoms in the fetus or neonate?

(1) Macrosomia in the fetus
(2) Delayed pulmonic maturity in the fetus
(3) Hypoglycemia in the newborn
(4) Hypocalcemia in the newborn

SUMMARY OF DIRECTIONS

A	B	C	D	E
1,2,3 only	**1,3 only**	**2,4 only**	**4 only**	**All are correct**

208. True statements about the twin-twin transfusion syndrome include which of the following?

(1) The donor twin develops hydramnios more often than the recipient twin
(2) Gross differences may be observed between donor and recipient placentas
(3) The donor twin usually suffers from a hemolytic anemia
(4) The recipient twin can develop widespread thromboses

209. The following statements about twins are true EXCEPT that

(1) perinatal mortality for twin fetuses is higher than that for singletons
(2) an increased risk of death for twins persists only for 1 month postpartum
(3) the perinatal mortality rate for monozygous twins is higher than that for dizygous twins
(4) intrauterine death from cord accidents are a rare cause of death in monoamniotic twins

210. An infant is likely to be compromised as a result of vaginal delivery that is accompanied by which of the following conditions?

(1) Prolapse of the umbilical cord
(2) Shoulder presentation
(3) Persistent brow presentation
(4) Persistent occiput posterior position

211. True statements describing toxoplasmosis in a pregnant woman include which of the following?

(1) It can be acquired by eating infected raw meat
(2) It occurs in 1 in every 2000 to 2500 pregnancies
(3) Infection in early pregnancy may lead to abortion
(4) Transplacental infection of the fetus is highly unlikely

212. The human placenta produces which of the following hormones?

(1) Gonadotropin
(2) Somatomammotropin
(3) Progesterone
(4) Hydrocortisone

213. Situations that increase the risk of morbidity or mortality for the fetus of a diabetic morther include

(1) maternal ketoacidosis
(2) maternal ketonuria in the absence of diabetic ketoacidosis
(3) maternal hyperglycemia
(4) maternal hypoglycemia

214. Chorioangiomas can be described by which of the following statements?

(1) They affect more than 5 percent of placentas
(2) They often are associated with anomalous cord insertions
(3) They often are associated with cords containing only two vessels
(4) They are the most common tumors of the placenta

215. Substances that cross the placenta poorly or not at all include

(1) thyroxine
(2) long-acting thyroid stimulator
(3) thyroid-stimulating hormone
(4) propylthiouracil

DIRECTIONS: The group of questions below consists of lettered choices followed by several numbered items. For each numbered item select the **one** lettered choice with which it is **most** closely associated. Each lettered choice may be used once, more than once, or not at all.

Questions 216–219

For each of the following substances, choose the mechanism of transplacental transport most likely to be employed.

(A) Simple diffusion
(B) Facilitated diffusion
(C) Active transport
(D) Pinocytosis
(E) None of the above

216. Carbon dioxide

217. Iron

218. Oxygen

219. Glucose

The Fetus, Placenta, and Newborn

Answers

189. The answer is C. *(Danforth, ed 4. pp 316–318.)* Streeter hypothesized that each organ system has a definite time for appearance and differentiation. Consequently, when an insult occurs, it cannot affect or alter a structure that has differentiated earlier or one that does not develop until after the insult is completed. Major heart and circulatory structures are found from 6 to 8 weeks postmenstrual age.

190. The answer is C. *(Pritchard, ed 16. p 573.)* The normal umbilical cord contains two arteries and one vein. The absence of one umbilical artery is found in less than 1 percent of all infants. Although the significance of a missing umbilical artery is somewhat controversial, absence of the artery may indicate that other congential anomalies also are present. Therefore, the obstetrician must verify the number of umbilical vessels and notify the pediatrician of any abnormality.

191. The answer is C. *(Burrow, ed 2. p 544.)* The incidence of pregnancy-induced hypertension seems to be decreased in women who smoke during pregnancy; this curious fact, which has yet to be explained, is supported by a number of epidemiological studies. Offspring of women who smoke more than five cigarettes daily from about the fourth month of pregnancy show decreases in birth weight of as much as 400 g when compared with matched controls.

The issue of premature delivery is a difficult one in that epidemiological studies reveal no overall downward shift in the distribution of gestational ages for infants of mothers who smoke; thus there appears to be a greater risk of true growth retardation rather than preterm delivery. However, there is a dose-related increase in the *proportion* of preterm babies born to women who smoke. These preterm deliveries account for a small proportion of total births so that the mean of gestational age distribution remains unchanged, yet these deliveries account for a large proportion of neonatal deaths. Therefore, while overall results show only a 0.02-week decrease in mean duration of pregnancy between smokers and non-smokers, the rate of delivery before 38 weeks is >7 per 1000 births for nonsmokers, 92 per 1000 for light smokers, and 116 per 1000 for heavy smokers.

192. The answer is A. *(Pritchard, ed 16. p 539.)* A pH of 7.20 to 7.24 is borderline abnormal and should be repeated within 30 minutes unless delivery intervenes. If the pH is less than 7.20, immediate collection of a confirmatory sample is necessary with movement toward prompt delivery if the low pH is continued; otherwise, labor may continue with repeat sampling periodically.

193. The answer is E. *(Burrow, ed 2. pp 450–451.)* Chronic alcohol abuse, which can cause liver disease, folate deficiency, and many other disorders in a pregnant woman, also can lead to the development of congenital abnormalities in the child. The chief abnormalities associated with the fetal alcohol syndrome are microcephaly, growth retardation, and cardiac anomalies. Chronic abuse of alcohol also may be associated with an incresed incidence of mental retardation in the children of affected women.

194. The answer is B. *(Aladjem, ed 2. pp 341–344.)* Deceleration of the fetal heart rate is related to hypoxia. Although fetal hypoxia also leads to a metabolic acidosis, which is reflected by low arterial pH and increased base deficits, deceleration of the fetal heart rate occurs before developement of the acidosis.

195. The answer is A. *(Pritchard, ed 16. pp 551–553.)* In circumvallate placenta, the thickened ring is a double fold of amnia and choria with degenerate decidua and fibra between. In a marginate placenta, decidua and fibra are interposed but the membranes are not folded. A degenerate placenta is a rare anomoly in which the central portion of the basal plate is absent and which may be mistaken for retention of a missing fragment in the uterus. Conversely, with succinturate placenta the accessory lobe may be inadvertantly retained in the uterus without detection.

196. The answer is D. *(Pritchard, ed 16, p 174.)* If a fetus weighs less than 500 g or is less than 20 weeks gestational age at delivery, an abortion, as opposed to a birth, is usually recorded for purposes of perinatal statistics. When a birth weight has not been obtained, a crown-rump length of 16 cm indicates a gestational age of 20 weeks. However, at 500 g, a fetus is more likely to have attained at least 22 weeks gestation with a crown-rump length of approximately 19 cm.

197. The answer is B (1, 3). *(Burrow, ed 2. pp 356–357.)* A suspicious genital lesion in pregnancy must be cultured for herpesvirus; if culture is positive, examination for lesions and cervical cultures are mandatory in the last month of pregnancy. Transplacental or ascending infection of the fetus with intact membranes are rare. Delivery by cesarean section is recommended for active lesions or positive culture within 2 to 4 weeks of delivery if membranes have been ruptured for less than 4 hours. Longer rupture probably exposes the fetus prior to delivery and abdominal delivery will not ensure safety. Conversely, with negative culture and absence of lesions, vaginal delivery can be undertaken with reasonable safety.

198.   The answer is D (4). *(Pritchard, ed 16. pp 639–640.)* Monozygotic twins are formed from the splitting of a single fertilized ovum and occur in approximately 1 birth in 250. Dizygotic twins, which are more common, result from multiple ovulations during the same menstrual cycle. The incidence of monozygotic twinning seems to be relatively constant despite differences in race, heredity, age, and hormonal therapy. Dizygotic twinning, on the other hand, is influenced by all of these factors; it occurs more commonly in blacks than in whites, seems to run (by the maternal-hereditary line) in families, and is more common with increasing age and parity. The use of clomiphene for ovulation induction is associated with multiple ovulation and an approximately 7 percent incidence of multiple gestation (as opposed to approximately 1.0 to 1.4 percent in the normal population). The use of gonadotropins to stimulate ovulation is associated with an even higher incidence of multiple gestations, with some series reporting as high as 40 percent.

199.   The answer is C (2, 4). *(Pritchard, ed 16. pp 185–187.)* Immunoglobulin G (IgG) easily crosses the placenta and thus is found in approximately equal amounts in maternal and fetal blood. Immunoglobulin M (IgM), on the other hand, is a large molecule and does not cross the placenta. Thus maternal levels of IgM are higher than fetal levels, unless and intrauterine infection causes the fetus to manufacture IgM. The gamma chains in hemoglobin (Hb) are what distinguish fetal hemoglobin from adult hemoglobin. Fetal hemoglobin (Hb F) contains two alpha and two gamma chains. Hb A, found in most adults, contains two alpha and two beta chains. One would therefore expect to find more gamma chains in the fetal blood than in maternal blood. Finally, cord-blood fibrinogen levels are normally quite low; maternal fibrinogen levels, on the other hand, are about 50 percent higher than levels in nonpregnant women.

200.   The answer is B (1, 3). *(Pritchard, ed 16. pp 949–952.)* Although all infants beyond 42 weeks gestation are considered postmature, the postmaturity syndrome does not affect all these infants. The syndrome itself consists of wasted subcutaneous tissues, peeling skin, long nails, diminished amniotic fluid, and meconium staining of amniotic fluid and baby. Prior to birth, ultrasound examination can detect a decreased amniotic fluid volume, and amniocentesis can be used to determine the presence or absence of meconium. The presence of postmaturity syndrome correlates with an increase in the stillbirth rate and an increase in neonatal complications, the most common of which are meconium aspiration and hypoglycemia. The incidence of cord entanglement also is increased, probably due to diminished amniotic fluid volumes. When gestation is prolonged beyond the forty-second week of pregnancy and meconium or oligohydramnios is present, prompt delivery should be performed.

201. The answer is A (1, 2, 3). *(Jeanty, pp 45, 55–67, 99–105.)* Determination of fetal age using biparietal diameter is most accurate before the 26th week when the rate of growth is faster and the variation among fetuses of the same age is less. Fetal death can be diagnosed by lack of limb or heart motion, irregularity of skull outline, or excessive flexion in posture. Polyhydramnios is characterized by increased uterine volume with extensive echo-free areas. Many neural tube defects and anencephaly can be diagnosed by abnormalities in the skull and spine on ultrasound.

202. The answer is D (4). *(Burrow, ed 2. pp 97–98.)* The lecithin-to-sphingomyelin (L/S) ratio, measured from amniotic-fluid samples, is a barometer of pulmonic maturity. If the L/S ratio is above whatever value denotes maturity in a particular laboratory, respiratory distress syndrome will probably not be present in the newborn. Lecithin seems to be involved in surfactant activity, and its secretion from the lungs into the amniotic fluid yields information about surfactant production in the fetal lungs. Amniotic-fluid creatinine values have been used to document fetal maturity; but because they also can reflect the muscle mass of a fetus, they are not as valid as the L/S ratio. The L/S ratio may reach maturity levels earlier in stressful situations, as in toxemia of pregnancy. Delay in pulmonic maturation occurs in association with mild diabetes but not with erythroblastosis fetalis.

203. The answer is A (1, 2, 3). *(Burrow, ed 2. pp 430–439.)* Fetal hydantoin syndrome is characterized by craniofacial anomolies, deficient growth, mental retardation, and limb defects. Valproic acid has been associated with increased risks of neural tube defects. Trimethadione-affected infants have developmental delay, low-set ears, palate anomolies, irregular teeth, V-shaped eyebrows, and speech disturbances. Although carbamazepine has been associated with hematological problems in patients, no reports of teratogenicity have been published. When possible, a seizure-free woman should be withdrawn from medication before pregnancy, but if she is actively epileptic, continued therapy is advised due to the danger of prolonged seizures.

204. The answer is A (1, 2, 3). *(Pritchard, ed 16. pp 476–477.)* The assessment tool for infants known as the Apgar score is based on the infant's condition 1 minute and 5 minutes after birth. Heart rate, respiratory effort, muscle tone, reflex irritability, and body color are assessed. The maximum score is 10 (2 points per category), and the lowest score is 0. A perfect score indicates heart rate greater than 100 beats per minute, good respiratory effort, active motion, vigorous crying, and pink body color. Responses that are present but not optimal earn a score of 1 per category, while an absence of response gives no score. Apgar scores of 4 to 7 at 1 minute indicate mild respiratory depression; infants who score under 4 are severely depressed. Thus, a low 1-minute Apgar score indicates the need for immediate resuscitation, and a low 5-minute Apgar score indicates increased risk of morbidity and mortality. The infant presented in the question is severely depressed, and the physician should assume nothing regarding resuscitation.

205. The answer is C (2, 4). *(Aladjem, ed 2. pp 56–62.)* Fetal heart rate has been shown to drop almost immediately when the umbilical circulation has been obstructed in experimental situations. This response is a reflex action that is caused by the sudden rise in central venous pressure and that disappears if the vagi are severed. A more prolonged obstruction of the umbilical circulation can cause a delayed fall in the fetal heart rate secondary to progressive asphyxia.

206. The answer is E (all). *(Burrow, ed 2. pp 333–346.)* A mild group B coxsackievirus infection of the mother during the antipartum period may give rise to a virulent infection in the newborn, sometimes resulting in a fatal encephalomyocarditis. A maternal rubella infection may cause neonatal hepatosplenomegaly, petechial rash, and jaundice; in addition, viral shedding may last for months or years. Herpes zoster, the causative agent of varicella (chickenpox), is an especially dangerous organism for the newborn. Varicella is rare in pregnancy, but if it occurs shortly before delivery, the viremia may spread to the fetus before protective maternal antibodies have had a chance to form. Congenital varicella can be fatal the the newborn; the increasing availability of zoster immunoglobulin, however, may allow clinicians to attack the infection before significant fetal viremia has developed. Herpesvirus can be acquired by the fetus as it passes down the genital tract and can cause a severe, often fatal herpes infection in the newborn.

207. The answer is E (all). *(Burrow, ed 2. pp 48–50.)* Maternal diabetes, especially of the milder classes, is associated with macrosomia in the fetus. Glucose crosses the placenta freely by facilitated diffusion, but insulin does not. The fetus, in response to the chronic glucose load, secretes increased quantities of insulin. Insulin acts as a growth hormone in the fetus, and the fetus becomes macrosomic. At delivery, the fetus is removed from the relatively glucose-rich maternal environment but continues to secrete increased amounts of insulin. Thus, the fetus may become hypoglycemic in the early hours of life unless early feedings, sometimes even intravenous glucose, is begun. Hypocalcemia may occur in as many as one-fourth of infants of diabetic mothers, possibly as a result of fetal parathyroid suppression stemming from maternal hypercalcemia. Lastly, fetal lung maturity, as measured by the lecithin-to-sphingomyelin ratio, may be delayed, especially in the infants of mothers who have mild diabetes.

208. The answer is C (2, 4). *(Benirschke, NY State J Med 61:4499, 1961.)* In the twin-twin transfusion syndrome, the doner twin is always anemic, due not to a hemolytic process but to the direct transfer of blood to the recipient twin. The recipient may suffer thromboses secondary to hypertransfusion and subsequent hemoconcentration. Although the donor placenta is usually pale and somewhat atrophied, that of the recipient is congested and enlarged. Hydramnios can develop in either twin but, because of circulatory overload, is more frequent in the recipient. Hydramnios when it occurs in the donor is due to congestive heart failure caused by severe anemia.

209. The answer is C (2, 4). *(Pritchard, ed 16. pp 652–653.)* The mortality rate for twins approaches that of singletons in the second year. Intertwining of umbilical cords is a common cause of death in monoamniotic twins.

210. The answer is A (1, 2, 3). *(Pritchard, ed 16. pp 806–820.)* Shoulder presentation, either as a transverse or an oblique lie, presents significant problems when vaginal delivery of an affected infant is attempted, because the shoulder is arrested by the margins of the pelvic inlet. Similarly, persistent brow presentation compromises the infant because the resultant extensive molding deforms the head. The presence of a prolapsed umbilical cord is also associated with significant compromise of infants delivered vaginally, since the cord becomes compressed between the presenting part and the margin of the pelvic inlet. Persistent occiput posterior position does not significantly compromise an infant during the course of a normal vaginal delivery.

211. The answer is B (1, 3). *(Pritchard, ed 16. pp 767–768.)* Toxoplasmosis, a protozoal infection caused by *Toxoplasma gondii*, can result from ingestion of raw or undercooked meat infected by the organism or from contact with infected cat feces. Its incidence in pregnant women is estimated to be 1 in every 150 to 700 pregnancies. Infection early in pregnancy may cause abortion; later in pregnancy, however, the fetus may become infected. A small number of infected infants develop involvement of the central nervous system or the eye; most infants who have the disease, however, escape serious clinical problems.

212. The answer is A (1, 2, 3). *(Pritchard, ed 16. pp 147–150, 162–164.)* The polypeptide hormones human chorionic gonadotropin (HCG) and human chorionic somatomammotropin (HCS) are produced by the syncytiotrophoblast of the human placenta. Because these hormones reflect placental rather than fetal integrity, the presence of HCG in the urine or blood may persist after fetal death (in the case of missed abortion) and even after spontaneous or therapeutic abortion. HCG is immunologically quite similar to pituitary luteinizing hormone (LH), the difference being in the amino acid sequence of the beta subunit. This fact must be considered when interpreting results of pregnancy tests based on HCG bioassay, results of which are not always positive until 42 days gestation. The specific immunoassay for the beta subunit of HCG, on the other hand, may be positive even before a menstrual period is missed. Progesterone is made in large amounts by the placenta. There is no good evidence to support a placental role in the production of adrenocorticosteroids.

213. The answer is A (1, 2, 3). *(Burrow, ed 2. p 50.)* Sophisticated management of high-risk diabetic individuals has reduced the incidence of diabetic ketoacidosis. When it occurs in pregnant women, however, it is associated with an extremely high fetal mortality rate. In addition, ketonuria in the absence of acidosis (i.e., starvation ketosis) has been correlated with decreased intelligence quotients in the offspring. Perinatal mortality has been correlated to hyperglycemia even in the absence of ketoacidosis, and this finding is the cornerstone of current recommendations urging strict control of diabetes during pregnancy. A correlation between maternal hypoglycemia and fetal morbidity or mortality has not been shown; in fact, rather severe episodes of hypoglycemia have been reported to have no effect on the outcome of pregnancy.

214. The answer is D (4). *(Aladjem, ed 2. p 284.)* Chorioangiomas are the most common placental tumor, occurring in approximately 1 percent of placentas. Despite attempts to correlate the presence of this tumor with hydramnios and fetal anomalies, no significant effect on fetal morbidity and mortality has been demonstrated, unless the size of the tumor is very great.

215. The answer is B (1, 3). *(Burrow, ed 2. pp 195, 204.)* Thyroxine crosses the placenta poorly, if at all. For this reason, a hyperthyroid mother does not transmit her hyperthyroidism to the fetus, and giving thyroid hormone to a hypothyroid mother will not raise fetal thyroxine levels significantly. Thyroid-stimulating hormone also does not cross to the fetus. On the other hand, propylthiouracil (PTU), an antithyroid drug, crosses easily and may suppress fetal thyroid function. Hyperthyroid women taking large doses of PTU therefore run the risk of having goitrous babies. Some clinicians, hoping to reverse the effect of PTU on the fetus, have given thyroxine to the mother; theoretically, however, this should not work, because the thyroid hormone should not get to the fetus. Long-acting thyroid stimulator (LATS) is present in many patients who have Grave's disease. Because LATS can cross the placenta, LATS levels should be obtained from such patients and the pediatrician should be alerted to possible neonatal thyrotoxicosis if LATS is present.

216–219. The answers are: 216-A, 217-C, 218-A, 219-B. *(Pritchard, ed 16. pp 180–182, 203–206.)* Oxygen travels from mother to fetus, and carbon dioxide from fetus to mother, by *simple diffusion* across the placenta. Carbon dioxide travels more rapidly than oxygen, probably because fetal and maternal blood have different affinities for these two substances. Iron is *actively transported* (i.e., in an energy-requiring process) from mother to fetus; as a result, the mother may become markedly iron-depleted during pregnancy, while the fetus does well. Glucose crosses to the fetus by *facilitated diffusion,* which means that its transfer across the placenta is more rapid than could be accounted for by simple diffusion alone. The fetus acts as a "glucose sink," continuously obtaining glucose at the expense of the mother. This fact may help to explain the lower-than-normal levels of maternal fasting blood glucose found during pregnancy. *Pinocytosis* describes the process by which liquid is imbibed by cells as a result of invagination of the cell membrane.

Pregnancy, Labor, Delivery, and Puerperium

DIRECTIONS: Each question below contains five suggested answers. Choose the **one best** response to each question.

220. Normal values for thyroid function tests increase during pregnancy in all of the following tests EXCEPT

(A) basal metabolic rate
(B) total thyroxine
(C) total triiodothyronine
(D) radioiodine uptake (percent)
(E) free thyroxine

Questions 221–223

The sketch shown below details the major landmarks of the fetal skull as it presents in the maternal pelvis. The perspective is that of the obstetrician facing the perineum.

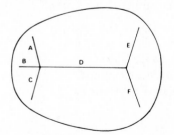

221. The position of the fetal vertex is

(A) left occiput anterior
(B) left sacrum transverse
(C) left occiput transverse
(D) right occiput transverse
(E) mentum posterior

222. The lambdoid sutures are

(A) **A** and **C**
(B) **A, C,** and **D**
(C) **B** and **D**
(D) **E** and **F**
(E) none of the above

223. The intersection of **D, E,** and **F** forms the

(A) caput succedaneum
(B) parietal prominence
(C) biparietal plane
(D) anterior fontanelle
(E) posterior fontanelle

224. The pH of amniotic fluid is

(A) 2.5 to 3.0
(B) 3.0 to 3.5
(C) 4.5 to 5.5
(D) 5.5 to 6.0
(E) 7.0 to 7.5

225. Which line on the echogram shown below represents the biparietal diameter of the fetal skull?

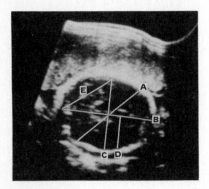

(A) Line **A**
(B) Line **B**
(C) Line **C**
(D) Line **D**
(E) Line **E**

226. A pregnant woman is seen 18 days after she has been exposed to rubella. Her hemagglutination inhibition titer is 1:8. Her physician should

(A) administer rubella vaccine
(B) recommend an abortion
(C) repeat the titer 2 days later
(D) repeat the titer 10 to 14 days later
(E) obtain weekly titers for the next 4 weeks

227. The oxytocin challenge test is considered negative if

(A) at least three uterine contractions occur in a 10-minute interval and late deceleration of fetal heart rate is absent
(B) at least three uterine contractions occur in a 10-minute interval and late deceleration is inconsistent
(C) less than three uterine contractions occur in a 10-minute interval, regardless of whether late deceleration occurs
(D) the uterus contracts at least once every 2 minutes, regardless of whether late deceleration occurs
(E) no uterine contractions are noted

228. The smallest anteroposterior diameter of the pelvic inlet is called the

(A) interspinous diameter
(B) true conjugate
(C) diagonal conjugate
(D) obstetric diameter
(E) none of the above

229. Which of the following agents cause uterine contractions?

(A) Ergotrate
(B) Oxytocin
(C) Methergine
(D) Prostaglandin E_2
(E) All of the above

230. A pregnant woman is discovered to be an asymptomatic carrier of *Neisseria gonorrhoeae*. A year ago, she was treated with penicillin for a gonococcal infection and developed a severe allergic reaction. Treatment of choice at this time would be

(A) tetracycline
(B) ampicillin
(C) erythromycin
(D) spectinomycin
(E) chloramphenicol

231. The major reason that birth-control pills are contraindicated for lactating mothers is their association with

(A) fibrocystic disease of the breast
(B) carcinoma of the breast
(C) thromboembolism in the newborn
(D) subsequent onset of juvenile diabetes
(E) jaundice in the newborn

---

232. A 25-year-old woman, gravida 1, para 0, who has a history of infertility, comes to your office at 20 weeks gestation. Her uterus is enlarged (24 weeks). She was treated in the past with a fertility drug, the name of which she does not know. You obtain an ultrasonogram, which is shown below. The most likely diagnosis is

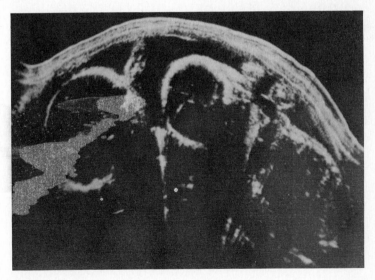

(A) hydatidiform mole
(B) placenta previa
(C) anencephalic fetus
(D) twins
(E) normal single-fetus pregnancy

233. The x-ray shown below, which was taken in the plane of the pelvic inlet, demonstrates which of the following types of pelvic morphology?

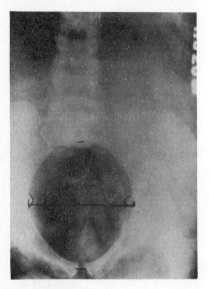

(A) Anthropoid
(B) Android
(C) Gynecoid
(D) Platypelloid
(E) Trianguloid

DIRECTIONS: Each question below contains four suggested answers of which **one or more** is correct. Choose the answer:

A	if	**1, 2, and 3**	are correct
B	if	**1 and 3**	are correct
C	if	**2 and 4**	are correct
D	if	**4**	is correct
E	if	**1, 2, 3, and 4**	are correct

234. The use of aspirin in pregnancy may be associated with which of the following complications?

(1) Polyhydramnios
(2) Maternal platelet dysfunction
(3) Premature labor
(4) Neonatal jaundice

235. True statements about $Rh_o(D)$ immune globulin (RhoGAM) include which of the following?

(1) Administration is therapeutically unsuccessful in approximately 1.5 percent of cases
(2) It should never be administered during pregnancy
(3) It usually is given in a dose of 300 μg within 72 hours of delivery of an Rh-positive infant to an unsensitized Rh-negative woman
(4) It can prevent ABO (blood group) incompatibility

236. Appropriate measures in the treatment of women who have edema of pregnancy include

(1) salt restriction
(2) weight control
(3) diuretics
(4) bed rest

237. Which of the following circumstances should alert an obstetrician to an increased likelihood of postpartum hemorrhage?

(1) Prolonged labor
(2) Rapid labor
(3) Oxytocin stimulation of labor
(4) Twin pregnancy

238. Advantages of the McDonald cerclage over the Shirodkar procedure to treat cervical incompetence include which of the following?

(1) A higher success rate is achieved
(2) There is less scarring of the cervix
(3) Nonabsorbable suture is used
(4) It is a technically easier procedure

239. In a lower uterine segment cesarean section, the advantages of a transverse incision as compared with a vertical incision include

(1) less blood loss
(2) less likelihood of extending the broad ligaments
(3) less likelihood of extending into the cervix and vagina
(4) more room for extraction of the fetus

240. True statements about the oxytocin challenge test (also called the contraction stress test) include which of the following?

(1) It determines the inducibility of the uterus
(2) Its effects are measured by internal monitors
(3) It is considered positive if the uterus contracts once every 2 minutes
(4) It can serve as a fetal stress test

241. The use of estrogen to suppress lactation is associated with which of the following?

(1) Venous thrombosis and thromboembolism
(2) Decreased prolactin levels
(3) Rebound breast engorgement
(4) Suppurative mastitis

242. Obstetrical analgesia and anesthesia can be described by which of the following statements?

(1) The most common cause of death due to anesthesia is pneumonitis from aspirated gastric material and juices
(2) Intravenous thiopental and other barbiturates are relatively ineffective in producing analgesia and can cause depression in the newborn infant
(3) Antacids given before general anesthesia can diminish the risk of serious pulmonary injury
(4) Naloxone, a narcotic antagonist, is effective only against respiratory depression induced by opioid narcotics

243. Electronic fetal monitoring is used to assess fetal well-being during labor. Patterns associated with fetal compromise include which of the following?

(1) Loss of beat-to-beat variability
(2) Late decelerations
(3) Persistent fetal tachycardia
(4) Variable decelerations

244. The use of which of the following antibiotics is contraindicated during pregnancy?

(1) Tetracycline
(2) Penicillin
(3) Chloramphenicol
(4) Ampicillin

DIRECTIONS: The group of questions below consists of lettered choices followed by several numbered items. For each numbered item select the **one** lettered choice with which it is **most** closely associated. Each lettered choice may be used once, more than once, or not at all.

Questions 245–249

The safety of immunization during pregnancy is a matter of concern and controversy that has prompted the American College of Obstetricians and Gynecologists to offer specific recommendations for the use of immunization therapy for pregnant women. For each disease vaccine listed below, select the recommendation with which it is most likely to be associated.

(A) Recommended if the underlying disease is serious
(B) Recommended after exposure or before travel to endemic areas
(C) Not routinely recommended but mandatory during an epidemic
(D) Contraindicated unless exposure to the disease is unavoidable
(E) Contraindicated

245. Poliomyelitis

246. Mumps

247. Influenza

248. Rubella

249. Hepatitis A

Pregnancy, Labor, Delivery, and Puerperium

Answers

220. The answer is E. *(Pritchard, ed 16. pp 250–251.)* Thyroid-binding globulin levels are increased in pregnancy. This is an effect of elevated levels of estrogen and is also seen in patients taking exogenous estrogens, such as oral contraceptives. Therefore there is an increase in total T4 and T3 along with a decrease in T3 resin uptake. Despite the increased total values of thyroid hormones, unbound or free, T4 and T3 values remain unchanged. There is a 25 percent increase in the basal metabolic rate. There is an increase in radioiodine uptake, but this test should not be performed in pregnancy because of the deleterious effects of radioactive iodine on the fetus.

221–223. The answers are: 221-C, 222-D, 223-E. *(Pritchard, ed 16. pp 176, 293–297.)* A good knowledge of the major landmarks of the fetal skull is essential for anyone performing deliveries. The position of the fetal vertex in the accompanying sketch is left occiput transverse. The lambdoid sutures (E and F) meet the sagittal suture (D) to form the posterior fontanelle. The occiput is just posterior to the posterior fontanelle. The posterior, or Y-shaped, fontanelle is the reference point for vertex presentations. The side of the maternal pelvis to which it is closest defines the position. The head is oriented in a transverse (or horizontal) manner, with the occiput nearest the maternal left side; thus, this is left occiput transverse. The anterior, or diamond-shaped, fontanelle, is made up of the intersection of the sagittal, frontal (B), and the two coronal (A and C) sutures. Extreme molding of the fetal head may make identification of these landmarks very difficult. Other clues to the position of the head include abdominal palpation of the back and small parts and, more important, palpation of an ear. If an ear can be felt and the relationship between the locations of the pinna and the auditory canal can be ascertained, the position of the vertex can be deduced.

224. The answer is E. *(Pritchard, ed 16. pp 407–408.)* The pH of amniotic fluid is generally 7.0 to 7.5. The pH of the vagina is 4.5 to 5.5. This distinction forms the basis of the nitrazine test to diagnose rupture of the membranes.

225. The answer is C. *(Pritchard, ed 16. p 345.)* The biparietal diameter is figured from the inner table of one area of the fetal skull (one echo) to the outer table of the other. In the echogram shown, the falx is easily seen in the midline. Therefore, line C represents the true biparietal diameters. Line A represents a diagonal from one table of the skull to another. Line B measures the longitudinal length of the skull. Line D represents the distance between the falx and the outer table of the fetal skull, and line E is a chord describing a portion of the circumference. The measurement of the biparietal diameter is essential to modern-day obstetricians because it can establish intrauterine gestational age.

226. The answer is D. *(Burrow, ed 2. pp 335–337.)* A titer of 1:8 obtained by a hemagglutination inhibition test may or may not indicate prior exposure to rubella virus. This titer in an exposed patient could represent a false positive result caused by the presence of nonspecific hemagglutinin inhibitors, which can be found in all human sera. On the other hand, a patient who has a titer of 1:8 18 days after exposure to rubella could be susceptible and harboring an inapparent infection that has just begun to stimulate manufacture of antibody. If a titer repeated 10 to 14 days later is the same as the first one, the patient is assumed to be immune. If, on the other hand, the repeat titer is 1:32 or greater, the initial titer most likely represented early antibody response to an inapparent infection. Rubella vaccination is contraindicated in pregnant women.

227. The answer is A. *(Pritchard, ed 16. pp 349–352.)* The oxytocin challenge test is negative if the uterus contracts at least three times in a 10-minute interval, if each contraction lasts 40 seconds or longer, and if the contractions are not accompanied by a late deceleration of the fetal heart rate. Test results should be considered suspicious if late deceleration is uneven and unsustained in spite of continuing uterine contractions. In the presence of hyperstimulation of the uterus, judged either by the contraction frequency (more than one every 2 minutes) or length (longer than 90 seconds), late deceleration of the fetal heart rate may not signify uteroplacental disease.

228. The answer is C. *(Pritchard, ed 16. p 279.)* The obstetric conjugate is the shortest distance between the prominatory of the sacrum and the symphysis pubis. It generally measures 10.5 cm. Because the obstetric conjugate cannot be clinically measured, it is estimated by subtracting 1.5 to 2.0 cm for the diagonal conjugate, which is the distance from the lower margin of the symphysis to the sacral prominatory. The true conjugate is measured from the top of the symphysis to the sacral prominatory. The interspinous diameter is the transverse measurement of the midplane and generally is the smallest diameter of the pelvis.

229. The answer is E. *(Pritchard, ed 16. pp 426–429.)* Oxytocin is an octopeptide secreted by the neurohypophysis. Parenterally administered oxytocin stimulates uterine contractions and is widely used to induce and augment labor. Ergotrate and methergine are alkaloid substances that are powerful stimulants of myometrial contractions. They are used after delivery to prevent and control postpartum hemorrhage but are too strong to use before delivery. Prostaglandin E_2 and F_2 are both capable of inducing and augmenting labor; however, in the United States neither is approved for use for these indications.

230. The answer is C. *(Monif, p 8.)* Erythromycin is the treatment of choice for pregnant women who have an asymptomatic *Neisseria gonorrhoeae* infection and who are allergic to penicillin. Although tetracycline also is an effective alternative to penicillin, its use is contraindicated in pregnancy. Spectinomycin is another drug effective in treating asymptomatic gonorrhea, but erythromycin is preferred in pregnant woman because of uncertain effects of spectinomycin on the fetus. Administration of chloramphenicol is not recommended to treat women, pregnant or not, who have cervical gonorrhea, and the use of ampicillin is contraindicated for penicillin-allergic patients.

231. The answer is E. *(Kase, p 1028.)* The synthetic sex steroids used in oral contraceptives may easily cross to the newborn in breast milk and cause jaundice in the newborn as well as other, as yet unrecognized effects. Other undesirable effects include suppression of lactation and increased risk of maternal thromboembolism in the early postpartum period. The pill has been associated with a decreased incidence of fibrocystic disease of the breast, but no association with breast cancer has been shown. Further, there is no known relationship to subsequent diabetes or an increase in thromboembolism in the newborn.

232. The answer is D. *(Pritchard, ed 16. pp 648–651.)* The ultrasonogram presented in the question clearly shows twins. The diagnosis can be made by noting the two heads (the circular densities). A hydatidiform mole would show no evidence of fetal parts or cranium. The presence of a spherical cranium rules out anencephaly. Because the placenta is anterior and superior, placenta previa is not present. Ultrasound has been very helpful in the diagnosis, early in gestation, of twins.

233. The answer is A. *(Pritchard, ed 16. pp 286–288.)* The anteroposterior diameter of the inlet of the anthropoid pelvis shown in the x-ray is greater than the transverse diameter. The anterior segment of an anthropoid pelvis is narrow, the ischial spines often are prominent, and the side walls may be somewhat convergent. In one American study, the anthropoid pelvis was found to be nearly twice as common (40 percent to 23 percent) in nonwhite women as in white women. This type of pelvis is far more likely than a gynecoid pelvis to be a source of dystocia.

234. The answer is C (2, 4). *(Pritchard, ed 16. p 322.)* Aspirin has been associated with platelet dysfunction and prolonged clotting times in both pregnant and nonpregnant individuals. Neonatal jaundice secondary to aspirin ingestion is caused by displacement of bilirubin from protein binding sites. The use of analgesic compounds that contain aspirin has also been associated with post dated gestations.

235. The answer is B (1, 3). *(Pritchard, ed 16. pp 963–965.)* $Rh_o(D)$ immune globulin (RhoGAM) is a concentrated sterile solution of human immunoglobulin G that contains anti-$Rh_o(D)$; it can prevent the formation of active $Rh_o(D)$ antibody in women, thereby impeding the development of Rh hemolytic disease of the newborn in subsequent deliveries. $Rh_o(D)$ immune globulin is usually given in an intramuscular dose of 300 μg within 72 hours of delivery. The failure rate, which is reported to be 1 to 2 percent, is attributed either to the development of sensitization in a subsequent pregnancy or to an unrecognized sensitization that already exists when the drug is administered. $Rh_o(D)$ immune globulin is of no benefit in ABO (blood group) incompatibility.

236. The answer is C (2, 4). *(Romney, p 687.)* Edema is present to a greater or lesser degree in all pregnant women but most frequently among women who gain an excessive amount of weight. Edema of pregnancy has traditionally been treated with salt restriction and diuretics; however, it is now clear that sodium and water retention are normal processes during pregnancy. More water than sodium is retained, so unnecessary salt restriction and diuretics may cause intravascular depletion. Diuretics also may cause sodium and potassium depletion in the mother. Thiazide diuretics have been implicated in hemorrhagic pancreatitis and deterioration of glucose tolerance in the mother and in thrombocytopenia in the newborn. The best treatment of edema of pregnancy is bed rest in the lateral recumbent position, which should improve renal perfusion, and weight control if obesity is the major problem.

237. The answer is E (all). *(Pritchard, ed 16. pp 877–879.)* Prolonged or rapid labor, oxytocin stimulation of labor, and twin pregnancy all predispose to uterine atony and, thus, to postpartum hemorrhage. A uterus that has required oxytocin in order to provide adequate labor is likely to need large amounts of oxytocin afterwards in order to stay contracted. A uterus that has stretched to accommodate twin gestations is likely to be atonic after it is emptied. No explanation is given for the clinical finding that a uterus that has been hypertonic and yielded a rapid labor is predisposed to atony.

238. The answer is C (2, 4). *(Pritchard, ed 16. pp 598–601.)* Of the several methods to treat cervical incompetence the McDonald and the Shirodkar cerclages are the two most commonly performed. The McDonald cerclage is accomplished by inserting a nonabsorbable suture in a purse-string fashion as high on the cervix as possible. With the Shirodkar cerclage the vaginal mucosa is incised anteriorly and posteriorly and the nonabsorbable suture is placed submucosaly to encircle the cervix. Of the two procedures, the McDonald technique is easier and causes less scarring. Success rates of both procedures are 85 to 90 percent.

239. The answer is B (1, 3). *(Pritchard, ed 16, p 1085.)* In a lower uterine segment cesarean section, a transverse incision results in less blood loss, because it goes through the thinned-out lower uterine segment and does not involve much of the myometrium, site of the large blood vessels. (However, if the placenta is implanted over the anterior lower uterine segment, blood loss can be significant.) The transverse incision also is less likely to extend into the cervix and vagina, because its direction of extension is usually horizontal. A transverse incision is more likely than a vertical incision to extend into the broad ligaments. If this happens, catastrophic hemorrhage can result. A vertical incision actually allows more room for extraction of the fetus, because it can extend upward toward the fundus. Many obstetricians prefer the vertical incision in situations where extra room is needed, as for example, in a breech presentation.

240. The answer is D (4). *(Pritchard, ed 16. pp 349–352.)* The oxytocin challenge test assesses the ability of the fetoplacental unit to withstand the stress of labor. After external monitors have measured the baseline activity of the uterus and fetal heart for 10 minutes, intravenous oxytocin is infused at a rate of 0.5 milliunits per minute. The rate is doubled every 15 to 20 minutes until three contractions, each of which last for 40 to 60 seconds, occur every 10 minutes. The test is considered positive if fetal heart rate consistently decelerates once uterine contractions have begun.

241. The answer is B (1, 3). *(Pritchard, ed 16. pp 918–919.)* Many agents have been used to suppress lactation in women who are not breast-feeding. Estrogens, both naturally occuring and synthetic compounds have been used alone or in combination with androgens. By decreasing antithrombin III levels, estrogen increases the risk of venous thrombosis and thromboembolism. Estrogens may increase prolactin levels. They block lactation at the level of the breast. Rebound engorgement can occur. There is no association of estrogens with suppurative mastitis.

242. The answer is E (all). *(Pritchard, ed 16. pp 435–442.)* In obstetrics, death from anesthesia most commonly results from pneumonitis caused by the inhalation of gastric acid. Administration of antacids before general anesthesia can lessen gastric acidity and therefore reduce the risk of serious pulmonary injury. The use of intravenous thiopental or other barbiturates, which are rather ineffective analgesics, can cause significant respiratory depression in the newborn. Narcotic antagonists, such as naloxone, levallorphan, and nalorphine, are effective only in reducing respiratory depression caused by opioid narcotics.

243. The answer is A (1, 2, 3). *(Pritchard, ed 16. pp 355–358.)* The types of uniform decelerations are generally described. Early decelerations (type I) are usually a benign pattern attributed to head compression. Late decelerations (type II) are often an ominous pattern indicating uteroplacental insufficiency causing fetal hypoxia. Persistent tachycardia may indicate a fetal response to hypoxia and compromise. Variable decelerations (type III) are not related to contractions and are usually associated with cord compression. Tachycardia is associated with febrile illness and, more rarely, fetal thyrotoxicosis. Beat-to-beat variability refers to the normal variation in time interval between successive r waves in the fetal ECG. Loss of beat-to-beat variability may also be indicative of fetal compromise.

244. The answer is B (1, 3). *(Monif, pp 19–26.)* Tetracycline may cause fetal dental anomalies and inhibition of bone growth if administered during the second trimester, and it is a potential teratogen to first-trimester fetuses. Tetracycline administration also can cause severe hepatic decompensation in the mother, especially during the third trimester. Chloramphenicol may cause the "gray baby" syndrome (symptoms of which include vomiting, impaired respiration, hypothermia, and, finally, cardiovascular collapse) in neonates who have received large doses of the drug. No notable adverse effects have been associated with the use of penicillin or ampicillin.

245–249. The answers are: 245-C, 246-E, 247-A, 248-E, 249-B. *(Pritchard, ed 16. p 321.)* The recommendations concerning immunization during pregnancy offered by the American College of Obstetricians and Gynecologists are as follows:

(1) Administration of influenza vaccine is recommended if the underlying disease is serious.

(2) Typhoid immunization is recommended when traveling to an endemic region.

(3) Hepatitis A immunization is recommended after exposure or before travel to developing countries.

(4) Cholera immunization should be given only to meet travel requirements.

(5) Tetanus–diphtheria immunization should be given if a primary series has never been administered or if 10 years have elapsed without receiving a booster.

(6) Immunization for poliomyelitis is mandatory during an epidemic but otherwise not recommended.

(7) Smallpox immunization is unnecessary since the disease has been eradicated.

(8) Immunization for yellow fever is recommended before travel to a high-risk area.

(9) Mumps and rubella immunizations are contraindicated.

(10) Administration of rabies vaccine is unaffected by pregnancy.

ABNORMALITIES
OF PREGNANCY

Spontaneous Abortion, Ectopic Pregnancies, and Trophoblastic Disease

DIRECTIONS: Each question below contains five suggested answers. Choose the **one best** response to each question.

250. The karyotype of a complete hydatidiform mole is

(A) 46,XY
(B) 45,X
(C) 46,XX
(D) 69,XXX
(E) none of the above

251. The most common complication of hypertonic saline abortion is

(A) hypofibrinogenemia
(B) hemorrhage
(C) amniotic fluid embolus
(D) retained placenta
(E) cervical laceration

Questions 252–254

A 19-year-old primigravid woman is expecting her first child; she is 12 weeks pregnant by dates. She has vaginal bleeding and an enlarged-for-dates uterus. In addition, no fetal heart sounds are heard. An ultrasound is obtained, as shown on the next page.

252. The most likely diagnosis of this woman's condition is

(A) sarcoma botryoides
(B) tuberculous endometritis
(C) adenocarcinoma of the uterus
(D) hydatidiform mole
(E) normal pregnancy

253. The safest and most reliable method for early diagnosis of this woman's condition is

(A) amniography
(B) ultrasonography
(C) abdominal roentgenogram
(D) pelvic arteriography
(E) human chorionic gonadotropin (HCG) titer

254. After uterine evacuation, management of the woman described above who has no clinical or radiographic evidence of metastatic disease should include

(A) weekly HCG titers
(B) hysterectomy
(C) single-agent chemotherapy
(D) combination chemotherapy
(E) radiation therapy

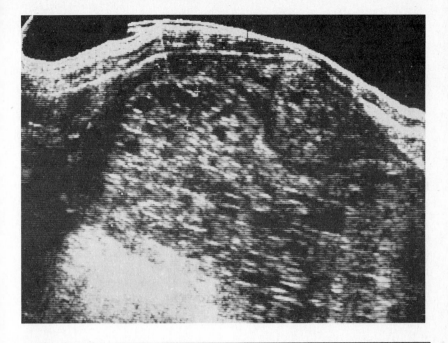

255. The most frequent pathogen currently implicated in infectious causes of early abortion is

(A) Brucella abortus
(B) Listeria monocytogenes
(C) Toxoplasma gondii
(D) Mycoplasma hominis
(E) Streptococcus agalacture

256. Habitual spontaneous abortion is defined as

(A) two or more abortions
(B) three or more consecutive abortions
(C) five or more abortions
(D) total of three abortions
(E) none of the above

257. All of the following have been suggested as a cause of habitual abortion in the first trimester EXCEPT

(A) luteal phase insufficiency
(B) maternal or paternal chromosomal abnormality
(C) anatomical uterine abnormalities
(D) psychiatric factors
(E) cervical incompetence

258. A woman previously delivered a normal infant and then during the next pregnancy aborted a fetus with a normal karyotype. The risk of spontaneous abortion with a subsequent pregnancy is

(A) 7 percent
(B) 24 percent
(C) 50 percent
(D) 90 percent
(E) none of the above

259. The chromosomal abnormality most often detected in first trimester abortuses is

(A) Turner syndrome
(B) polyploidy
(C) autosomal monosomy
(D) autosomal trisomy
(E) unbalanced translocation

260. Which of the following findings is most commonly associated with ectopic pregnancy?

(A) Abnormal menstrual history
(B) Negative urine pregnancy test
(C) Abdominal pain
(D) Positive test for the Bsubunit of human chorionic gonadotropin
(E) Adnexal mass on pelvic examination or sonography

261. A 32-year-old woman, gravida 3, para 3, presents with abdominal pain. Her last menstrual period was 6 weeks ago, and a pregnancy test is positive. The specimen shown below is obtained at laparotomy. The most likely diagnosis is

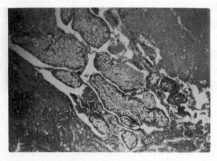

(A) incomplete abortion
(B) missed abortion
(C) hydatidiform mole
(D) tubal ectopic pregnancy
(E) none of the above

262. A 19-year-old woman comes to the emergency room and reports that she had passed out at work earlier in the day. She has mild vaginal bleeding, and her abdomen is diffusely tender and distended. In addition, she complains of shoulder and abdominal pain. Temperature is 36.4°C (97.6°F); pulse rate, 120 per minute; and blood pressure, 96/50 mmHg. To confirm the diagnosis suggested by the available clinical data, which of the following diagnostic procedures would best be utilized?

(A) A pregnancy test
(B) Posterior colpotomy
(C) Dilatation and curettage
(D) Culdocentesis
(E) Laparoscopy

263. A patient has been successfully operated on for an ectopic pregnancy. Preoperative laboratory studies return and reveal that she is Rh negative. She had 8 weeks of amenorrhea prior to her surgery. Which of the following statements regarding this patient is true?

(A) There is no need to give Rhogam
(B) Rhogam 300 mg should be administered
(C) MicroRhogam 50 mg should be administered
(D) An antibody titer should be obtained, and if it is negative the appropriate amount of Rhogam should be administered.
(E) Rhogam should be administered according to the outcome of the Kleihauer-Betke smear.

264. Which of the following statements correctly applies to ectopic pregnancy?

(A) The Arias-Stella reaction is diagnostic of ectopic pregnancy

(B) Interstitial ectopic pregnancies generally rupture later, bleed more severely, and are usually more difficult to diagnose than isthmic or ampullary pregnancies

(C) Isthmic ectopic pregnancies are the most common

(D) Most ectopic pregnancies can be diagnosed sonographically by detecting a fetal sac in the adnexal region, outside the uterine cavity

(E) Tubal abortions do not cause significant intraperitoneal hemorrhage

DIRECTIONS: Each question below contains four suggested answers of which **one or more** is correct. Choose the answer:

A	if	**1, 2, and 3**	are correct
B	if	**1 and 3**	are correct
C	if	**2 and 4**	are correct
D	if	**4**	is correct
E	if	**1, 2, 3, and 4**	are correct

265. Indications for instituting single-agent chemotherapy following evacuation of a hydatidiform mole usually include

(1) a rise in HCG titers
(2) a plateau of HCG titers for 3 successive weeks
(3) failure of HCG titers to return to normal 8 weeks after evacuation
(4) appearance of liver or brain metastases

266. True statements about interstitial tubal pregnancy include which of the following?

(1) Its incidence increases in women who have had a salpingectomy
(2) It tends to rupture at an earlier stage than other tubal pregnancies
(3) A significant percentage can be diagnosed before rupture
(4) Rupture causes less blood loss than rupture of pregnancies in the ampullary portion of the tube

267. Criteria that are especially reliable in determining a patient's response to chemotherapy for gestational trophoblastic disease include

(1) duration of the disease
(2) urine levels of HCG
(3) sites of metastases
(4) the patient's age

268. Observations on the role of actinomycin D and methotrexate in the management of gestational trophoblastic disease suggest that

(1) resistance to one agent results in cross-resistance to the other
(2) actinomycin D is safer than methotrexate for women whose liver function is impaired
(3) there is no additive effect in combining the two agents
(4) actinomycin D is as effective as methotrexate for primary treatment

269. Disorders referred to as gestational trophoblastic disease include

(1) hydatidiform mole
(2) chorioadenoma destruens
(3) choriocarcinoma
(4) ovarian choriocarcinoma

270. Determination of the presence of a growing tumor in a patient who has gestational trophoblastic disease could be established by

(1) serial chest x-rays
(2) evaluation of menstrual function
(3) presence of lactation
(4) serial HCG titers

Spontaneous Abortion, Ectopic Pregnancies, and Trophoblastic Disease

Answers

250. The answer is C. *(Pritchard, ed 16. p 559.)* The karyotype is believed to derive from a paternal haploid that duplicates to the 46,XX status. Partial moles with a concomitant fetus are often triploid (69,XXX or 69,XXY).

251. The answer is D. *(Pritchard, ed 16. p 608.)* Retained placenta occurs in approximately 13 percent of all saline abortions. Hypofibrin ogenemia is commonly associated with saline abortions but actually occurs quite rarely (0.3 percent).

252. The answer is D. *(Jeanty, pp 213–215. Romney, ed 2. pp 1094–1097.)* The history, clinical picture, and a tissue sample of the woman described in the question are characteristic of hydatidiform mole. The most common initial symptoms include an enlarged-for-dates uterus and continuous or intermittent bleeding in the first two trimesters. Other symptoms include hypertension, proteinuria, and hyperthyroidism. Hydatidiform mole is ten times as common in the Far East as in North America, and it occurs more frequently in women over 45 years of age. A tissue sample would show a villus with hydropic changes and no vessels. Grossly, these lesions appear as small, clear clusters of grapelike vesicles, the passage of which confirms the diagnosis.

253. The answer is B. *(Sciarra, ed 2, vol 4, chap 48, pp 1–27.)* Ultrasonography is the safest and the most reliable method for early diagnosis of hydatidiform mole. Amniography, although another accurate method, requires percutaneous insertion of a needle into the uterine cavity and injection of a radiopaque contrast dye, which carries a risk of radiation exposure to a normal fetus. An abdominal roentgenogram cannot demonstrate a hydatidiform mole; however, if a fetal skeleton is visualized, it is unlikely that a hydatidiform mole also exists since coexisting molar and fetal pregnancies are rare. Elevated human chorionic gonadotropin (HCG) titers are not diagnostic. Pelvic arteriography would expose an accompanying normal fetus to high doses of radiation.

254. The answer is A. *(Sciarra, ed 2, vol 4, chap 48, pp 1–27.)* The condition of women who have hydatidiform moles but no evidence of metastatic disease should be followed routinely after uterine evacuation by HCG titers. Most authorities agree that prophylactic chemotherapy should not be employed in the routine management of women having hydatidiform moles, because 85 to 90 percent of affected patients will require no further treatment. For a young woman in whom preservation of reproductive function is important, surgery is not routinely indicated.

255. The answer is D. *(Pritchard, ed 16. p 590.)* There have been increased investigations linking *Mycoplasma* infections with early abortions. There may be a role for preconceptual tetracycline therapy in couples with histories of habitual abortions.

256. The answer is B. *(Pritchard, ed 16. p 587.)* Although there is an increased tendency to begin work-up for habitual abortion after two consecutive abortions, the definition is still considered to be three or more consecutive abortions.

257. The answer is E. *(Pritchard, ed 16. pp 597–599.)* Although all these factors have been suggested as causes of habitual abortion, cervical incompetence rarely if ever presents itself before the 16th week of pregnancy. Anatomical abnormalities may present either as first or second trimester losses, depending in part upon the degree of abnormality.

258. The answer is B. *(Pritchard, ed 16, p 597.)* Since the abortus was normal and a previous infant was normal, the etiology of the abortion is more likely to have been an abnormality of the mother, which will persist with the next pregnancy. With an abnormal fetal karyotype in the abortus, the risk would be 7 percent.

259. The answer is D. *(Thompson, ed 3. pp 162–163.)* A number of investigators have detected a high frequency of chromosomal abnormalities by tissue culture of first trimester abortuses. The frequency of these abnormalities is about 36 percent, of which approximately 45 percent are autosomal trisomies, 25 percent are polyploidies, and 20 percent are 45,XO. The remaining 10 percent include autosomal monosomies, structural abnormalities, and mosaics.

260. The answer is D. *(Pritchard, ed 16. pp 535–549.)* All these findings may be associated with extrauterine pregnancy, but the extremely sensitive radioimmunoassay for the Bsubunit of human chorionic gonadotropin is so sensitive that it is virtually always positive in these cases. Unfortunately, this test is *not* diagnostic of the condition.

261. The answer is D. *(Sciarra, ed 2, vol 6, chap 29, pp 1–6.)* The photomicrograph accompanying the question shows villi within a tubular structure; the villi are easily identified by the presence of cytotrophoblasts. The diagnosis is tubal ectopic pregnancy. Molar pregnancy, incomplete abortion, and missed abortion also can be associated with the presence of villi, but specimens from these disorders would not be obtained at laparotomy.

262. The answer is D. *(Kistner, ed 3. pp 305–308. Pritchard, ed 16. pp 539–540.)* The clinical history presented in this question is a classic one for a ruptured tubal pregnancy accompanied by a hemoperitoneum. Because pregnancy tests are negative in almost 50 percent of cases, they are of little practical value in an emergency. Dilatation and curettage would not permit rapid enough diagnosis, and the results obtained by this procedure are variable. Posterior colpotomy requires an operating room, surgical anesthesia, and an experienced operator with a scrubbed and gowned associate. Refined optic and electronic systems have improved the accuracy of laparoscopy, but this new equipment is not always available, and the procedure requires an operating room and, usually, surgical anesthesia. Culdocentesis is a rapid, nonsurgical method to confirm the presence of unclotted, intraabdominal blood from a ruptured tubal pregnancy.

263. The answer is C. *(ACOG Tech Bull 61:3, 1981.)* Ectopic pregnancies are capable of producing Rho(D) sensitization, therefore RhIg should be used. Prior to 13 weeks, 50 mg RhIg appears adequate to prevent sensitization.

264. The answer is B. *(Pritchard, ed 16. pp 527–534.)* Ectopic pregnancies most commonly occur in the ampullary portion of the fallopian tube. When they do occur in the interstitial portion of the tube (2.5 percent of cases), they are harder to diagnose, may rupture late because of the thick myometrium into which they grow, and often lead to severe, life-threatening hemorrhage because of the tremendous vascularity of the area. The histologic finding of an Arias-Stella reaction suggests abnormal pregnancy but is *not* diagnostic of ectopic gestation. Ultrasound examination is most useful in indirectly ruling out ectopic pregnancy by demonstrating an intrauterine gestation, as coexistence of a second ectopic pregnancy is extremely rare. Even tubal abortion can lead to severe intraperitoneal bleeding.

265. The answer is A (1, 2, 3). *(Romney, ed 2. pp 1098–1099.)* Single-agent chemotherapy usually is instituted if levels of HCG have remained elevated 8 weeks after evacuation of a hydatidiform mole. Approximately 50 percent of the patients who have persistently high HCG titers will develop malignant sequelae. If HCG titers rise or reach a plateau for 2 to 3 successive weeks following molar evacuation, a single-agent chemotherapy should be instituted, provided that the trophoblastic disease has not metastasized to the liver or brain. The presence of such metastases usually requires initiation of combination chemotherapy.

266. The answer is B (1, 3). *(Mattingly, ed 5. pp 376–377.)* Rupture of an interstitial tubal pregnancy can cause severe blood loss, because this area is supplied by both uterine and ovarian vessels. Serious shock usually ensues rapidly. Because interstitial tubal pregnancies usually rupture at a later stage than other tubal pregnancies, a significant percentage can be diagnosed before rupture. Women who have had salpingectomies are at increased risk for interstitial pregnancy, and it has been suggested that salpingectomy by too vigorous a cornual wedge resection is the cause.

267. The answer is A (1, 2, 3). *(DiSaia, ed 2. pp 196–196.)* Women who have had gestational trophoblastic disease for less than 4 months, whose 24-hour urine titers of HCG are less than 100,000 IU, and whose metastases are limited to the vagina or lungs have a 95-percent cure rate and are thus considered low-risk patients. Patients whose disease has lasted for more than 4 months, whose HCG titer is greater than 100,000 IU per 24 hours, and who have liver or brain metastases, on the other hand, are classified as high-risk patients.

268. The answer is C (2, 4). *(DiSaia, ed 2. pp 200–211.)* The first successful treatment regimen for women who had gestational trophoblastic disease consisted of single-agent methotrexate chemotherapy. Subsequent studies combining methotrexate, actinomycin D, and an alkylating agent were successful in treating methotrexate-resistant trophoblastic disease. Actinomycin D, then studied as a single agent, proved to be as effective as methotrexate; in addition, it was not hampered by cross-resistance in methotrexate-resistant tumors and was safer to use in women who have impaired liver function.

269. The answer is A (1, 2, 3). *(Romney, ed 2. pp 1093–1094.)* The term gestational trophoblastic disease refers to a group of neoplasms — that is, hydatidiform mole, choriocarcinoma, and chorioadenoma destruens — that are characterized by the histological degeneration of the gestational trophoblast. Although the pregnancy itself can be affected (e.g., hydatidiform mole), neoplasms of this group also can be diagnosed following normal intrauterine pregnancies, ectopic pregnancies, or abortions. Chorioadenoma destruens is a molar lesion that has invaded the myometrium; choriocarcinoma, which can occur anywhere in the uterus, is composed of malignant trophoblastic cells that metastasize easily. The term gestational trophoblastic disease is preferred because these neoplasms are often managed without a precise histological diagnosis. The presence or absence of metastases is more important in determining prognosis and treatment.

270. The answer is D (4). *(Romney, ed 2. pp 1093–1094.)* Viable trophoblastic tissue produces HCG; therefore, the presence of elevated HCG titers confirms the amount of functioning trophoblastic tissue and thus the size of the tumor. Monitoring serial HCG titers allows the physician to determine not only the need for chemotherapy but also its effectiveness. Theca-lutein cysts tend to decrease in size following evacuation of a hydatidiform mole despite the persistence of viable trophoblastic cells; and normal cyclic menstruation may reappear in spite of continued disease activity. Chest x-ray changes often persist for several months after HCG titers have returned to normal.

Medical, Surgical, and Obstetrical Complications of Pregnancy

DIRECTIONS: Each question below contains five suggested answers. Choose the **one best** response to each question.

271. A 24-year-old woman appears at 8 weeks of pregnancy and reveals a history of pulmonary embolism 7 years ago during her first pregnancy. She was treated with intravenous heparin followed by several months of oral Coumadin and has had no further evidence of thromboembolic disease for over 6 years. Which of the following statements about her current condition is true?

(A) Having no evidence of disease for over 5 years means that her risk of thromboembolism is not greater than normal
(B) Impedence plethysmography is not a useful study to evaluate her for deep venous thrombosis in pregnancy
(C) Doppler ultrasonography is not a useful technique to evaluate her for deep venous thrombosis in pregnancy
(D) The patient should be placed on low-dose heparin therapy throughout her pregnancy and the puerperium
(E) She is at highest risk for recurrent thromboembolism during the second trimester of pregnancy.

272. The most common cause of death in women who have eclampsia is

(A) ruptured liver
(B) acute renal failure
(C) cerebral hemorrhage
(D) pulmonary embolism
(E) septic shock

273. A 17-year-old primigravida at 37 weeks gestation appears on the delivery floor with a blood pressure of 170/120, 3 proteinuria, 4 deep tendon reflexes, and 3 pretibial hand and facial edema. Appropriate management includes all of the following EXCEPT

(A) CBC, BUN, creatinine, liver function tests, platelet count, coagulation profile.
(B) intravenous or intramuscular therapy with magnesium sulfate
(C) induction of labor after rapid stabilization
(D) intravenous Apresoline (hydralazine) immediately for persistent BP elevation
(E) amniocentesis for lecithin/sphingomyelin ratio

110

274. Respiratory depression from magnesium sulfate overdose generally occurs at a serum level above

(A) 2 mg/L
(B) 4 mg/L
(C) 6 mg/L
(D) 8 mg/L
(E) 10 mg/L

Questions 275–277

A 24-year-old primigravid woman develops spider angiomata, palmar erythema, and diffuse pruritus at 28 weeks gestation. You obtain a set of liver function tests, which reveal the following serum levels: alkaline phosphatase, 190 IU/L (normal: 21–91 IU/L); glutamic oxaloacetic transaminase, 38 IU/L (normal: 6–18 IU/L); total bilirubin, 1.8 mg/100 ml (normal: 0.3–1.0 mg/100 ml); direct bilirubin, 1.0 mg/100 ml (normal: 0.1–0.3 mg/100 ml).

275. What is the most likely diagnosis of this woman's condition?

(A) Cirrhosis
(B) Infectious hepatitis
(C) Cholestasis
(D) Acute pancreatitis
(E) Cholecystitis

276. The most appropriate treatment would be

(A) observation
(B) bed rest and high-protein diet
(C) oral corticosteroids
(D) low-fat diet
(E) oral cholestryamine

277. After delivery, the physician should advise the woman to

(A) avoid further pregnancies
(B) avoid high-fat foods
(C) avoid oral contraceptives
(D) have a cholecystectomy
(E) none of the above

278. All of the following statements about autoimmune thrombocytopenic purpura (ATP) in pregnancy are true EXCEPT that

(A) platelet production is normal or greater in the bone marrow
(B) bleeding time may be normal because of the presence in the circulation of young, hyperactive platelets
(C) peripheral destruction of antibody-coated circulating platelets may result in abnormally low maternal platelet counts
(D) cesarean section may not always prevent fetal hemorrhage
(E) a maternal platelet count about 100,000/mm^3 at the time of delivery ensures safety for the newborn

279. Which of the following statements about wound dehiscence following cesarean section is NOT true?

(A) Vertical abdominal incisions more commonly dehisce than transverse incisions
(B) Mass closures of the abdominal wall significantly decrease the risk of dehiscence
(C) The incidence of dehiscence is lower following cesarean section than following cholecystectomy
(D) There are no clearcut diagnostic signs of dehiscence short of exploring the wound surgically
(E) Asthma significantly increases the risk of dehiscence

280. The initial maternal immunological response to a primary rubella infection is the elaboration of

(A) immunoglobulin M
(B) immunoglobulin G
(C) immunoglobulin A
(D) immunoglobulin D
(E) complement-fixation antibodies

281. Which of the following statements is true about placental abruption?

(A) Coagulopathy results from the consumption of clotting factors by the tetroplacental clot
(B) More than 50 percent of patients with this condition develop significant hypofibrinogenemia (less than 150 mg/dl)
(C) Less than 10 percent of patients with this condition develop significant hypofibrinogenemia (less than 150 mg/dl)
(D) Vigorous fluid, blood, and electrolyte replacement is generally adequate to prevent severe renal failure
(E) Many patients require dialysis despite vigorous fluid, blood, plus electrolyte replacement

282. Which of the following statements concerning placenta previa is true?

(A) Its incidence decreases with maternal age
(B) Its incidence is unaffected by parity
(C) The initial hemorrhage is painless and rarely fatal
(D) Management no longer includes a "double set-up"
(E) Bleeding is usually painful

283. Which of the following statements about placenta previa is true?

(A) Consumptive coagulopathy is a frequent complication
(B) The first episode of hemorrhage is generally severe enough to warrant immediate delivery
(C) Most cases of placenta previa diagnosed sonographically at the 22d week of gestation will never present as clinical problems
(D) Abdominal delivery is contraindicated if the fetus is dead
(E) With modern techniques, "double set-up examination" is an obsolete procedure

284. Viremia and the presence of rubella virus in the throat of infected individuals bear which of the following relationship to the onset of the rubella rash?

(A) They precede the rash by 5 to 7 days
(B) They precede the rash by 1 to 2 days
(C) They occur coincidentally with the rash
(D) They occur 1 to 2 days after the rash
(E) They bear no consistent relationship to the onset of the rash

285. For patients developing preeclampsia in their first pregnancy, which of the following is an associated future risk?

(A) Diabetes mellitus
(B) Chronic hypertension
(C) Habitual abortion
(D) Chronic liver disease
(E) Increased risk of third trimester stillborns in subsequent pregnancies

286. Although rheumatic heart disease is becoming less common, it still occurs during pregnancy. Deteriorating cardiac status in a pregnant woman is most likely to be associated with

(A) aortic regurgitation
(B) aortic stenosis
(C) mitral regurgitation
(D) mitral stenosis
(E) tricuspid regurgitation

287. The most common cause of uterine rupture during pregnancy is

(A) previous myomectomy
(B) previous cesarean section
(C) external trauma
(D) transverse lie
(E) oxytocin stimulation of labor

DIRECTIONS: Each question below contains four suggested answers of which **one or more** is correct. Choose the answer:

A	if	**1, 2, and 3**	are correct
B	if	**1 and 3**	are correct
C	if	**2 and 4**	are correct
D	if	**4**	is correct
E	if	**1, 2, 3, and 4**	are correct

288. Women who have systemic lupus erythematosus should be counseled that

(1) pregnancy is contraindicated, because it will exacerbate the disease
(2) if pregnant, they should have a therapeutic abortion to prevent a progression of their symptoms
(3) their disease is likely to inhibit their fertility
(4) their disease is likely to flare up after delivery

289. True statements about hyperthyroidism in pregnancy include which of the following?

(1) Affected women may be treated with thiourea compounds
(2) It is harder to control in pregnant than in nonpregnant women
(3) It may cause neonatal thyrotoxicosis
(4) It is an indication for interrupting a pregnancy

290. Pregnant women who have diabetes mellitus are affected more often than nondiabetic women by which of the following conditions?

(1) Preeclampsia and eclampsia
(2) Infection
(3) Postpartum hemorrhage after vaginal delivery
(4) Hydramnios

291. A 29-year-old Rh-negative woman (gravida 5, para 4) is 18 weeks pregnant. Her last child had erythroblastosis fetalis and required four exchange transfusions at birth. The father of her current pregnancy is not the father of her other children. Although he is Rh positive, he is a heterozygote. True statements regarding this case include which of the following?

(1) The infant has a 75 percent chance of being born with erythroblastosis fetalis
(2) The woman should be followed with serum titers, and amniocentesis should be performed when the titers are two dilutions greater than baseline values
(3) If fetal hydrops is demonstrated ultrasonographically or amniographically, intrauterine transfusions should be performed prior to 20 weeks gestation
(4) O-negative blood that has been crossmatched against the mother's serum should be used for an intrauterine transfusion, if a transfusion is indicated

292. Erythroblastosis fetalis can be caused by maternal incompatibility with which of the following fetal erythrocyte antigens?

(1) Kell
(2) Kidd
(3) Duffy
(4) Lewis

293. Pregnancy-induced hypertension is associated with which of the following lesions?

(1) Periportal hemorrhages
(2) Ischemic lesions
(3) Large subcapsular hematomas
(4) Primary fibrin deposits in hepatic arterioles

294. Pregnancy should be strongly discouraged in women who have

(1) artrial septal defect
(2) ventrical septal defect
(3) patent ductus arteriosus
(4) Eisenmenger syndrome

295. Pregnancy has which of the following effects on diabetic women?

(1) Tendency toward ketoacidosis during early pregnancy
(2) Tendency toward hyperglycemia during early pregnancy
(3) Increase in insulin requirement during early pregnancy
(4) Increase in insulin requirement during late pregnancy

296. Hypothyroidism can be characterized by which of the following statements?

(1) It is uncommon during pregnancy
(2) It is associated with an increased abortion rate
(3) It is associated with an increased stillbirth rate
(4) It is genrally improved by pregnancy

297. If polyhydramnios is suspected, which of the following maternal conditions must be ruled out?

(1) Rh isoimmunization
(2) Systemic lupus erythematosus
(3) Diabetes mellitus
(4) Congential heart disease

298. True statements about hypoparathyroidism in pregnancy include which of the following?

(1) Its etiology is most commonly iatrogenic
(2) It is best treated with oral calcium and vitamin D
(3) It is a contraindication to breast-feeding
(4) It is associated with a marked increase in spontaneous abortions

299. Ovarian neoplasms of pregnant women can be characterized by which of the following statements?

(1) They are usually malignant
(2) They are most often confined to one ovary
(3) They may spread transplacentally to the fetus
(4) They can be mistaken for a cystic corpus luteum

SUMMARY OF DIRECTIONS

A	B	C	D	E
1,2,3 only	1,3 only	2,4 only	4 only	All are correct

300. A 27-year-old woman (gravida 3, para 2) comes to the delivery floor at 37 weeks gestation. She has had no prenatal care. She complains that, on bending down to pick up her 2-year-old child, she experienced sudden, severe back pain. This pain now has persisted for 2 hours. Approximately 30 minutes ago she noted bright red blood coming from her vagina. By the time she arrives at the delivery floor, she is contracting strongly every 3 minutes; the uterus is quite firm even between contractions. By abdominal palpation the fetus is vertex with the head deeply engaged. Fetal heart rate is 130 beats per minute. The fundus is 38 cm above the symphysis. Blood for clotting is drawn, and a clot forms in 4 minutes. Clotting studies are set to the laboratory. The initial course of action would be

(1) stabilize maternal circulation
(2) administer oxytocin to stimulate labor
(3) insert a intrauterine catheter for fetal monitoring
(4) administer heparin immediately

301. True statements about appendicitis during pregnancy include which of the following?

(1) Premature labor occurs commonly
(2) Mortality rate is much higher in pregnant than nonpregnant women
(3) Symptoms may be mistaken for those classically associated with pregnancy itself
(4) It is frequently mistaken for pyelitis of the right kidney

302. Maternal hyperparathyroidism can be characterized by which of the following statements?

(1) Diagnosis is made more often after pregnancy than during pregnancy
(2) Neonatal tetany may result
(3) Incidence of pathological fractures is increased
(4) Fertility, labor, and delivery are adversely affected

303. In infected women, cytomegalovirus can be recovered from

(1) saliva
(2) urine
(3) cervical secretions
(4) liver biopsy specimens

304. True statements about pregnancy-induced hypertension include which of the following?

(1) The incidence varies widely around the world
(2) Women who have had hypertension of pregnancy once have a 10 percent chance of developing it in a later pregnancy
(3) Elevations in systolic or diastolic blood pressures may be diagnostically significant even at blood pressure values less than 140/90 mmHg
(4) Young primiparous women have the lowest incidence

305. Premature separation of the placenta occurs more commonly than normal in association with which of the following conditions?

(1) Previous abruptio placentae
(2) Chronic hypertension
(3) Pregnancy-induced hypertension
(4) Delivery of twins

306. Nausea and vomiting are common in pregnancy. Hyperemesis gravidarum, however, is a much more serious and potentially fatal problem. Findings that should alert the physician to the diagnosis of hyperemesis gravidarum *early* in its course include

(1) electrocardiographic evidence of hypokalemia
(2) weight loss
(3) jaundice
(4) ketonuria

307. Common findings in the incompetent cervix syndrome include

(1) painless dilatation of the cervix
(2) a history of cervical trauma
(3) spontaneous rupture of the membranes at midpregnancy
(4) recurrent miscarrage at 14 to 16 weeks gestation

DIRECTIONS: The groups of questions below consist of lettered choices followed by several numbered items. For each numbered item select the **one** lettered choice with which it is **most** closely associated. Each lettered choice may be used once, more than once, or not at all.

Questions 308–310

For each clinical situation that follows, select the most likely placental disorder.

(A) Placenta accreta
(B) Placenta circumvallata
(C) Placenta membranacea
(D) Placenta succenturiata
(E) Vasa praevia

308. A 24-year-old woman, gravida 2, para 1, goes into premature labor at 33 weeks gestation after an apparently normal antepartum course

309. An apparently normal pregnancy culminates in the spontaneous delivery of an infant who weighs 3.2 kg (7 lb) with Apgars 9/9. The placenta delivers spontaneously followed by an unusual amount of uterine bleeding

310. After the low forceps delivery of an infant who weights 1.8 kg (4 lb) to a 27-year-old woman, gravida 4, para 3 (whose second baby was born by cesarean section due to fetal distress but whose third baby delivered vaginally), the placenta does not deliver spontaneously. After 20 minutes the obstetrician attempts a manual removal but is unable to identify a plane of cleavage

Questions 311–313

For each patient described, choose the diagnostic category (according to the Priscilla White classification) that is most appropriate.

(A) Normal
(B) Class A diabetic
(C) Class B diabetic
(D) Class C diabetic
(E) Class D diabetic

311. The patient is a 17-year-old primigravid woman who was diagnosed as being diabetic at age 9 and is currently taking 30 units of Lente insulin every morning. She is 18 weeks pregnant

312. The patient is a 26-year-old woman, gravida 3, para 2. Her first baby weighed 4.1 kg (9 lb). A glucose tolerance test is done at 28 weeks gestation after 2 days of carbohydrate loading; the test dose is 100 g of oral glucose. Blood sugars (mg/100 ml) are measured as follows: fasting, 88; 1-hour, 179; 2-hour, 144; 3-hour, 123

313. The patient is a 22-year-old primigravid woman who has a strong family history of diabetes. About 6 months before becoming pregnant, she had a glucose tolerance test. Although test results were abnormal, she was told that the results indicated chemical diabetes only and that no treatment was necessary. She has never been in ketoacidosis and has no symptoms now. An oral glucose tolerance test given at 28 weeks gestation (same method as described in question 312) reveals the following levels (mg/100 ml): fasting value, 92; 1-hour, 170; 2-hour, 148; 3-hour, 127

Questions 314–317

For each description that follows, select the microorganism with which it is most likely to be associated.

(A) Rubella virus
(B) Cytomegalovirus
(C) Group A β-hemolytic streptococci
(D) Group B β-hemolytic streptococci
(E) *Toxoplasma gondii*

314. This organism may cause epidemics of puerperal sepsis

315. A pregnant woman may become infected with this organism by contact with infected cat feces

316. An effective vaccine exists for the prevention of adult infection with this organism

317. This organism is an important cause of neonatal sepsis and meningitis

Questions 318–322

For each description that follows, select the disorder with which it is most likely to be associated.

(A) Placental polyps
(B) Placenta previa
(C) Abruptio placentae
(D) Ectopic pregnancy
(E) Spontaneous abortion

318. Associated with the Arias-Stella phenomenon

319. Premature placental separation

320. Associated with maternal hypertension

321. May be due to defective vascularization of the decidua caused by inflammation or atrophy

322. Usually accompanied by thickened placental villi, hemorrhage into the decidua basalis, and evidence of necrosis in tissues near the bleeding

Medical, Surgical, and Obstetrical Complications of Pregnancy

Answers

271. The answer is D. *(Burrow, ed 2. pp 172–183.)* Patients with a history of thromboembolic disease in pregnancy are at high risk to develop it in subsequent pregnancies. Impedence plethysmography or doppler ultrasonography are useful techniques even in pregnancy, and should be done as baseline studies. Patients should be treated prophylactically with low-dose heparin therapy through the postpartum period as this is the time of highest risk of this disease.

272. The answer is C. *(Burrow, ed 2. pp 13–22. Romney, ed 2. p 688.)* Preeclampsia, a disease of pregnancy, is characterized by hypertension, edema, and proteinuria after the 20th week of gestation. If not properly treated, preeclampsia may progress to eclampsia with accompanying convulsions and coma. Cerebral hemorrhage is the most common cause of death in women who have eclampsia. Sixty percent of women who die 2 days or less after the onset of convulsions are found subsequently to have cerebral hemorrhages. Evidence suggests that the pathophysiology of the lesions involves cerebral vasoconstriction. The maternal mortality rate from eclampsia is 3 to 5 percent; the fetal mortality rate is 17 to 20 percent.

273. The answer is E. *(Pritchard, ed 16. pp 681–684.)* Because severe preeclampsia is a disease that can be complicated by vascular, renal, hematologic, and hepatic disease, as well as a coagulopathy, laboratory studies to evaluate these possibilities are needed. Thereafter, prevention of seizures with a medication like magnesium sulfate and control of unstable hypertension should be undertaken. After initial stabilization, induction of labor should begin in order to terminate the pregnancy causing the disease. In a patient beyond the 37th week of pregnancy, there is no need to assess the state of fetal pulmonic maturity, especially when severity of the preeclampsia places mother and intrauterine fetus at jeopardy.

274. The answer is E. *(Pritchard, ed 16. p 692.)* Magnesium levels of 6 to 8 mg/L fall within the therapeutic range of this anticonvulsive medication. Deep tendon reflexes disappear at 9 to 10 mg/L, and levels above this may lead to respiratory depression. Levels about 12 mg/L run the risk of cardiac depression.

275–277. The answers are: 275-C, 276-E, 277-C. *(Pritchard, ed 16, pp 757–759.)* The most likely diagnosis for the woman described in the question is cholestatic jaundice of pregnancy (cholestasis). Spider angiomata and palmar erythema are normal occurrences in pregnant women and do not imply hepatic disease. Generalized pruritus in pregnancy, however, may be caused by cholestasis. In this disorder, bilirubin may or may not be elevated and elevation, if present, is usually mild. Although serum alkaline phosphatase levels may double during normal pregnancy, they are usually even higher in cholestasis of pregnancy. If placental (heat-stable) alkaline phosphatase can be distinguished from the hepatic isozyme, then hepatic alkaline phosphatase will show an increase in patients with cholestasis. Levels of serum glutamic-oxaloacetic transaminase may be mildly elevated.

The appropriate treatment for this condition, if the itching is intractable, is oral cholestyramine, an exchange resin that ties up bile salts in the gastrointestinal tract and presumably reduces their levels in the periphery. Although its safety in pregnancy is not unequivocally established, oral cholestyramine is commonly used for this condition when treatment is necessary.

Cholestasis tends to recur in subsequent pregnancies and to accompany use of oral contraceptives. If the patient is willing to go through another pregnancy with the symptoms described, it is not contraindicated; however, oral contraceptives are probably a poor choice for family planning in these patients. In the case described, there is no reason to suspect pancreatitis; cirrhosis is not exacerbated by pregnancy; the enzyme values do not support hepatitis; and the patient does not show symptoms of cholecystitis.

278. The answer is E. *(Burrow, ed 2. pp 74–76.)* ATP is an immunologic disorder wherein antibodies to an individual's own platelets lead to peripheral destruction of these cells by the reticuloendothelial system, thus leading to reduced numbers of circulating platelets. Platelets continue to be produced in greater than normal numbers, leading to large numbers of active young platelets in the circulation that may function to keep the bleeding time close to normal. Because maternal IgG antibody may cross the placenta, coating fetal platelets and leading to thrombocytopenia in the fetus, an atraumatic delivery should be accomplished to protect the fetus. Unfortunately, even cesarean section may not offer complete protection, as at least one case of neonatal hemorrhage and death following cesarean section has been reported. Maternal platelet counts above 100,000 do *not* guarantee adequate fetal counts.

279. The answer is D. *(Sciarra, ed 2, vol 1, chap 56, pp 7–10; chap 57, pp 9–10.)* Vertical upper abdominal incisions carry the greatest risk of dehiscence. Following cesarean section, this complication is most common in patients with pulmonary disease that leads to excessive coughing postoperatively, thereby straining the wound excessively. Drainage of serosanguinous fluid from the incision beyond the first 24 postoperative hours is said to be pathognomonic of wound dehiscence.

280. The answer is A. *(Burrow, ed 2. p 337.)* The first response to a primary infection of rubella and other viruses is the elaboration of immunoglobulin M (IgM). Although IgM, once produced, is present for at least several weeks, rising levels of immunoglobulin G (IgG) account for the fact that IgG eventually comprises nearly all antibody detected in the serum. Complement-fixation antibodies usually appear 7 to 10 days after appearance of the rubella rash.

281. The answer is D. *(Pritchard, ed 16. p 501.)* Thirty percent of abruptions resulting in fetal death also result in significant hypofibrinogenemia. The mechanism of the coagulopathy is most likely *not* just the consumption of clotting factors by the retroplacental clot, but rather a disseminated intravascular coagulation. When severe hemorrhage occurs, there is definite risk of acute renal failure. This complication can be prevented through vigorous fluid, blood, and electrolyte replacement, thereby avoiding the need for dialysis.

282. The answer is C. *(Pritchard, ed 16. pp 513–514.)* The initial hemorrhage in placenta previa is usually painless and rarely fatal. If the fetus is premature and if hemorrhaging is not severe, vaginal examination of a woman suspected of having placenta previa frequently can be delayed until 37 weeks of gestation; this delay in the potentially hazardous examination reduces the risk of prematurity, which often is associated with placenta previa. Vaginal examination, when needed to determine whether a low-lying placenta is covering the internal os of the cervix, should be performed in an operating room fully prepared for an emergency cesarean section (i.e., a "double set-up"). Increasing maternal age and multiparity are associated with a higher incidence of placenta previa.

283. The answer is C. *(Pritchard, ed 16. pp 508–513.)* Unlike abruptio placentae, placenta previa is rarely complicated by coagulopathy. Most often the first episode of bleeding is relatively mild but should alert the physician to the possible diagnosis. Up to 45 percent of patients undergoing ultrasound examination in the 2nd trimester may have low lying placentas, but the majority of these migrate from the cervical os by the third trimester. Despite fetal loss, cesarean section may be needed to prevent further maternal hemorrhage. The double-setup examination still has a place in obstetrics.

284. The answer is A. *(Burrow, ed 2. p 335.)* Both viremia and the excretion of virus from the throats of individuals infected with rubella occur 5 to 7 days before the appearance of the characteristic maculopapular rash. The importance of this relationship is that by the time a pregnant woman first notes the appearance of a rash on one of her children, she already has been exposed to the disease and may, in fact, be infected. If one member of a family develops rubella, all other members who are susceptible to the disease usually become infected.

285. The answer is A. *(Pritchard, ed 16. pp 694–695.)* Careful long-term follow-up studies of preeclamptic women have failed to reveal long-term hypertensive disease. However, Chesley et al. showed diabetes to be 2.5 to 4 times more common in previously preeclamptic women than controls. When patients with chronic hypertension are removed from these studies, pure preeclampsia seems to have little other long-term risk.

286. The answer is D. *(Burrow, ed 2. pp 155–157.)* Nearly all of the circulatory changes that normally accompany pregnancy are harmful to a woman who has mitral stenosis. Left atrial pressure rises because of increased cardiac output and shortened diastolic filling time; as a result, pulmonary flow is accentuated. Atrial fibrillation may occur suddenly during pregnancy, and pulmonary edema may supervene. Cardioversion may be necessary to reverse atrial fibrillation. Mitral regurgitation is unlikely to be worsened by pregnancy, although prophylaxis for subacute bacterial endocarditis would be indicated for affected women. Aortic stenosis is unusal as a pure lesion; associated problems, if they are going to develop at all, are most likely to develop in the immediate postpartum period, when rapid volume shifts can occur. Aortic regurgitation also is rare as pure lesion and again is most likely to cause problems just after delivery.

287. The answer is B. *(Pritchard, ed 16, pp 861–863.)* More than any other factor, delivery by cesarean section in an earlier pregnancy predisposes a woman to uterine rupture in subsequent pregnancies. Oxytocin stimulation of labor also is associated with rupture of the uterus and, in fact, may be the second most common cause. Other factors associated less frequently with uterine rupture include previous myomectomy, external trauma (such as an accident or bullet wound), breech delivery, and congenital or acquired defects of the uterus.

288. The answer is D (4). *(Burrow, ed 2. pp 481–487. Pritchard, ed 16. pp 768–769.)* Studies of the effect of pregnancy on the course of systemic lupus erythematosus (SLE) have been inconsistent in their findings. Some studies suggest a worsening of the disease, while others show remission or no effect at all. If a woman who is informed that her lupus might get worse during pregnancy still wants to have a child, she may be supported in her plans. Women should be advised to await a clinical remission of the disease before attempting pregnancy, since the course of SLE is more favorable when pregnancy occurs during such a remission. In most cases therapeutic abortion is not indicated, because the postpartum flare-up, especially in renal disease, may occur whether the pregnancy has been terminated by abortion or delivery. For some very sick patients, however, abortion may be lifesaving. Only in cases involving severe renal disease does lupus seem to decrease the fertility rate.

289. The answer is B (1, 3). *(Burrow, ed 2. pp 202–209.)* Hyperthyroidism in pregnancy may cause neonatal thryotoxicosis. The mechanism is not the transmission of triiodothyronine or thyroxine to the baby, but rather the crossing of long-acting thyroid stimulator (LATS) to the baby with subsequent hyperfunction of the fetal thyroid gland. Not all hyperthyroid women have LATS; and it is only those who do who are at risk for neonatal thyrotoxicosis. The usual treatment for hyperthyroidism in pregnancy is administration of thiourea compounds, although in some centers surgery is popular. Hyperthyroidism often becomes less severe during pregnancy, especially during the last trimester, at which time requirements for thiourea drugs often decrease. Because hyperthyroidism is a treatable disorder, it is not an indication for terminating a pregnancy.

290. The answer is E (all). *(Pritchard, ed 16. p 743.)* Maternal diabetes mellitus can affect a pregnant woman and her fetus in many ways. The development of preeclampsia or eclampsia is about four times as likely as among nondiabetic women. Infection also is more likely not only to occur but also to be severe. The incidence of fetal macrosomia or death and of dystocia are increased; and hydramnios is common. The likelihood of postpartum hemorrhage after vaginal delivery and the frequency of cesarean section both are increased in diabetic women.

291. The answer is D (4). *(Queenan, ed 2. pp 12–14, 27–44, 149–267.)* An Rh-negative woman married to a heterozygous Rh-positive man has a 50 percent chance of having an Rh-positive baby. Spectrophotometric analyses of the woman's amniotic fluid should be performed to detect bilirubin pigment; they should begin at 22 to 23 weeks gestation and be repeated every 2 weeks until delivery. (Serum titers are very inaccurate in women who were sensitized in previous pregnancies.) If the level of bilirubin pigment suggests imminent fetal demise, intrauterine transfusion of the pulmonically immature fetus is indicated. Tranfusion before 23 to 24 weeks gestation should not be attempted because of technical difficulties and the extremely poor chance of success at so early a stage. When intrauterine transfusions are performed, O-negative blood that is crossmatched against the mother's serum should be used.

292. The answer is A (1, 2, 3). *(Pritchard, ed 16. pp 972–973.)* Erythroblastosis fetalis, also known as isoimmune hemolytic disease of the newborn, results from the transplacental passage of maternal blood-group antibodies and subsequent destructive reaction with fetal erythrocyte antigens. It is theoretically possible for any blood-group antigen with the exceptions of Lewis and I antigens to cause erythroblastosis fetalis. Lewis and I antigens are not present on fetal red blood cells; furthermore, the antibodies to these two antigens are immunoglobulin M, which does not cross the placenta.

293. The answer is A (1, 2, 3). *(Romney, pp 687–688.)* Pregnancy-induced hypertension is associated with two types of hepatic lesions: periportal hemorrhages, which eventually are supplanted by fibrin deposits, and ischemic lesions, which can vary greatly in size and severity. It has been hypothesized that it is the spasm of hepatic arterioles, and not the primary deposition of fibrin, that is responsible for the hemorrhagic lesions.

294. The answer is D (4). *(Burrow, ed 2. p 160.)* Eisenmenger's syndrome consists of severe pulmonary hypertension combined with a bidirectional or reversed shunt through a patent ductus arteriosus or an atrial or ventrical septal defect. The death rate during pregnancy for women who have this syndrome is higher than in any other form of congenital heart disease. Death usually occurs at or just after delivery and is probably associated with a sudden drop in peripheral vascular resistance. Atrial and ventricular septal defects, in the absence of pulmonary hypertension and right-to-left shunting, rarely cause problems during pregnancy. Unless shunting is minimal, a patent ductus arteriosus is usually detected by the time a woman becomes pregnant. Again, only reversal of the shunt should pose any problems.

295. The answer is D (4). *(Burrow, ed 2. pp 45–46.)* Although during early pregnancy the diabetogenic effects of placental hormones are not marked, there is still a net transfer of glucose from mother to fetus. For this reason, there is a tendency toward maternal hypoglycemia rather than hyperglycemia; ketoacidosis is rare and insulin reactions are common. In fact, one of the first symptoms of pregnancy in a diabetic woman may be hypoglycemia and decreasing insulin need. Later on in pregnancy, however, insulin requirements increase markedly and are about two-thirds higher than before pregnancy. Hypoglycemia now becomes less of a problem than ketoacidosis.

296. The answer is A (1, 2, 3). *(Burrow, ed 2. pp 195–199.)* It is not known why hypothryoidism is uncommon during pregnancy; however, the most widely supported explanation is that many hypothyroid patients are anovulatory and thus do not easily become pregnant. However, if a hypothyroid patient does become pregnant, her disease, if untreated, could lead to abortion and stillbirth. For this reason, most perinatologists prefer to treat hypothyroidism vigorously during pregnancy. For example, if a woman who has been placed on low-dose thyroid replacement for poorly documented hypothyroidism becomes pregnant, administration of thyroid hormone probably should be increased to full replacement dose for the remainder of the pregnancy; after delivery, hormone therapy should be discontinued in order to reevaluate thyroid function.

297. The answer is B (1, 3). *(Pritchard, ed 16. pp 578–579.)* Polyhydramnios is defined as the presence of more than 2000 ml of amniotic fluid. This volume of amniotic fluid results in a tense uterus with a size greater than expected with a left mentoposterior position (LMP) and a fetus that is difficult to outline on palpation. Twin pregnancies (especially monozygotic twins), maternal diabetes mellitus, Rh isoimmunization or any other cause of erythroblastosis fetalis, and congenital anomalies of the fetus, especially gastrointestinal and central nervous system anomalies, are all associated with an increased incidence of polyhydramnios. There is no increased association with maternal systemic lupus erythematosus (SLE) or maternal heart disease.

298. The answer is A (1, 2, 3). *(Burrow, ed 2. pp 230–232.)* Hypoparathyroidism is most commonly iatrogenic, occurring when the parathyroid glands have been inadvertently removed at the time of thyroidectomy. The disease is characterized by low levels of serum calcium and high levels of serum phosphate. The usual treatment is oral calcium and vitamin D. Hypoparathyroid mothers should not breast-feed their children, because the calcium drain of breast-feeding may worsen their hypocalcemia. The outcome of pregnancy in the hypoparathroid patient who is under treatment should be excellent. If tetany occurs during pregnancy, hypoparathyroidism should be suspected, especially if the patient has had previous thyroid surgery; the most common cause of tetany during pregnancy, however, is alkalosis.

299. The answer is C (2, 4). *(DiSaia, ed 2. 439–443.)* Ovarian neoplasms associated with pregnancy are usually benign; only 3 to 6 percent are found to be malignant. The neoplasms are most often unilateral when malignant. It has been estimated that 10 percent of ovarian masses discovered during pregnancy represent an enlarged, cystic corpus luteum. Transplancental spread of ovarian carcinoma to the fetus has not been documented.

300. The answer is B (1, 3). *(Pritchard, ed 16. pp 495–508. Romney, ed 2. pp 675–676.)* The patient described in the question presents with a classic history for abruption—that is, the sudden onset of abdominal pain accompanied by bleeding. Physical examination reveals a firm, tender uterus with frequent contractions, which confirms the diagnosis. The fact that a clot forms within 4 minutes suggests that coagulopathy is not present. Because abruption is often accompanied by hemorrhaging, it is important that appropriate fluids (i.e., lactated Ringer's solution and whole blood) be administered immediately to stabilize the mother's circulation. Cesarean section may be necessary in the case of a severe abruption, but only when fetal distress is evident or delivery is unlikely to be accomplished vaginally. Internal monitoring equipment should provide an early warning that the fetus is compromised. The internal uterine catheter provides pressure recordings, which are improtant if oxytocin stimulation is necessary. Generally, however, patients with abruptio placentae are contracting vigorously and do not need oxytocin.

301. The answer is E (all). *(Mattingly, ed 5. pp 409–413.)* Pregnancy and appendicitis share many of the same signs and symptoms, including nausea, vomiting, abdominal discomfort, constipation, and leukocytosis. Because urinary tract symptoms are associated commonly with appendicitis of pregnant women, the disease also can be mistaken for pyelitis. Maternal mortality rates and fetal prematurity are increased in women who are pregnant and have appendicitis.

302. The answer is A (1, 2, 3). *(Burrow, ed 2. pp 228–230.)* Hyperparathyroidism, which is caused by a parathyroid adenoma, is characterized by elevated levels of serum calcium and symptoms associated with hypercalcemia. These symptoms include weakness, nausea, polyuria, and polydipsia; renal stones and pathological fractures also can occur. Because the milder of these symptoms may be seen in normal pregnancies, the presence of hyperparathryodism may be missed during pregnancy. More than half of the infants born to hyperparathyroid mothers have neonatal tetany – the first clue, in many instances, to the fact that the mother has the disease. The tetany is due to hypocalcemia in the newborn and occurs usually at 5 to 14 days of age. Hyperparathyroid patients do not have increased infertility problems. Labor and delivery are usually normal; however, the incidence of small-for-dates infants is increased.

303. The answer is E (all). *(Burrow, ed 2. pp 340–341.)* Cytomegalovirus can be recovered from the urine, saliva, cervical secretions of infected women, and specimens from a liver biopsy. Urine is the best source for recovering cytomegalovirus, which may be present in concentrations as high as 1 million virus particles per milliliter. Cultures of the virus, which is slow-growing, may not be positive until a month or more has passed.

304. The answer is B (1, 3). *(Burrow, ed 2. pp 13–16.)* Worldwide, the incidence of pregnancy-induced hypertension varies from a low of 2 percent in the Far East to almost 30 percent in Puerto Rico. Peak incidences occur in two groups: young primiparous women and multiparous women who are older than 35 years of age. Moreover, women who have had hypertension of pregnancy in the past have a 33 percent chance of developing the disease again in later pregnancies. Because of the difficulty in defining normal blood pressures for pregnant women, elevations in the systolic component of 20 mmHg or more or the diastolic component of 10 mmHg or more during pregnancy are defined as abnormal, notwithstanding the absolute blood pressure values. The terminology regarding hypertension in pregnancy is still in flux. The most inclusive term is hypertensive states of pregnancy. This is recommended by the American College of Obstetrics and Gynecology Committee on Terminology for general use. If the hypertension was not present before conception, then pregnancy-induced hypertension is also acceptable, but the term toxemia has fallen into disfavor.

305. The answer is E (all). *(Pritchard, ed 16. pp 495–508.)* Premature separation of the placenta (abruptio placentae) occurs in approximately 1 percent of all deliveries. Previous abruptio placentae, chronic hypertension, and pregnancy-induced hypertension all predispose to premature separation of the placenta. The placenta also is more likely than normal to separate between the birth of a first and second twin. Clinically, the severity of abruption ranges from a minimal amount of vaginal bleeding and rapid labor to massive hemorrhage, shock, consumptive coagulopathy, and fetal death. Clinical signs of abruption include an irritable, tender uterus, an enlarging uterus, hypertonic labor, and abdominal pain. Vaginal bleeding may or may not be present; in fact, some of the most severe abruptions with coagulopathies occur with "concealed hemorrhage," in which the retroplacental clot is contained within the uterus and has no egress to the vagina.

306. The answer is C (2, 4). *(Burrow, ed 2. pp 259–260.)* Hyperemesis gravidarum is intractable vomiting of pregnancy and is associated with disturbed nutrition. Early signs of the disorder include weight loss, up to 5 percent of body weight, and acetonuria. Because vomiting causes potassium loss, electrocardiographic evidence of potassium depletion, such as inverted T waves and prolonged Q-T and P-R intervals, is usually a later finding. Jaundice also is a later finding and probably is due to fatty infiltration of the liver; occasionally acute hepatic necrosis occurs. Hypokalemic nephropathy with isosthenuria may occur late. Hypoproteinemia also may result, caused by poor diet as well as by albuminuria. Patients who have hyperemesis gravidarum are best treated (if the disease is early in its course) with parenteral fluids and electrolytes, sedation, rest, vitamins, and antiemetics if necessary. In some cases, isolation of the patient is necessary. Very slow reinstitution of oral feeding is permitted after dehydration and electrolyte disturbances are corrected. Therapeutic abortion may be necessary in rare instances; usually, however, the disease improves spontaneously as pregnancy progresses.

307. The answer is A (1, 2, 3). *(Pritchard, ed 16. pp 598–601.)* When an incompetent cervix is suspected, weekly cervical examinations beginning at 16 to 18 weeks gestation can reveal evidence of cervical dilatation or effacement in time to perform corrective surgery. The most commonly used techniques are the Shirodkar cervical suture (cerclage), in which the purse-string suture is buried under the vaginal mucosa and the bladder pushed back for higher placement of the stitch, and the McDonald cervical suture, a simple purse-string suture most widely used when the cervix is well effaced. Once the diagnosis has been made, a cerclage procedure may be performed prophylactically in subsequent pregnancies, prior to any change in the cervix. This is best done at 14 to 16 weeks, well past the time when spontaneous abortion is common. Because it is not until 16 to 18 weeks that the fetus begins to occupy the lower uterine segment, it would be unlikely that incompetent cervix would be the cause of recurrent pregnancy loss at 14 to 16 weeks.

308–310. The answers are: 308-B, 309-D, 310-A. *(Pritchard, ed 16. pp 124, 551, 553, 574, 575, 884–888.)* A circumvallate placenta contains a grayish-white ring located a variable distance from the edge of the placenta. The membranes (amnion and chorion) are folded over at this ring and are not in contact with the substance of the placenta peripheral to the ring. The fetal vessels do not go beyond the ring. Placenta circumvallata is associated with an increased rate of prematurity; why the rate is increased is unknown.

A succenturiate placenta is characterized by an accessory lobe apart from the main body of the placenta. Fetal vessels usually course through the membranes between the main and accessory lobes and can be identified on inspection of the membranes. If the fetal vessels on their way between the lobes should pass over the cervix, vasa praevia occurs. This condition is potentially dangerous, because the membranes may rupture, in turn rupturing a fetal vessel and causing fetal hemorrhage. If a succenturiate lobe is left within the uterus after the main body of the placenta has been delivered, postpartum hemorrhage can result; therefore, the presence of an accessory lobe should be checked for by intrauterine exploration.

Placenta accreta is a condition in which the usual plane of cleavage (Nitabuch's layer) between the placenta and decidua is absent and the villi attach to the myometrium. It is more common in women who have uterine scars, such as in the patient described in the question, and who have undergone previous cesarean section. Complications of placenta accreta are in part iatrogenic. An overly vigorous attempt at manual removal may cause uterine inversion or perforation and severe bleeding. A hysterectomy may be necessary, although leaving the placenta in place and treating the patient with methotrexate may suffice. Severe complications are most common with the more severe forms of placenta accreta. These forms are known as placenta increta, if the villi grow into the muscle of the uterus, and placenta percreta, if the placenta grows through the myometrium.

311–313. The answers are : 311-E, 312-A, 313-B. *(Burrow, ed 2. pp 42–45.)* The Priscilla White classification is the most widely used descriptive categorization of diabetes in pregnant women. To a certain extent, as the classes progress alphabetically, the fetal prognosis becomes increasingly poor. A class A diabetic patient is one who either is diagnosed during pregnancy and needs no insulin or, if diagnosed before pregnancy, was asymptomatic and needed no treatment. A class B diabetic patient is overtly diabetic and was diagnosed after the age of 20; in addition, the duration of the disease is less than 10 years. A class C diabetic women was diagnosed either between the ages of 10 and 20 years or from 10 to 20 years ago. Diagnosis of a class D diabetic women was made either before the age of 10 or more than 20 years ago.

The normal values for a glucose tolerance test during pregnancy differ from those of nonpregnant women. With 2 days of carbohydrate loading and a 100 g oral glucose tolerance test, a patient, to be considered diabetic, must exceed two of the following four blood-sugar values (mg/100 ml): fasting, 90; 1-hour, 165; 2-hour, 145; 3-hour, 125. If serum or plasma levels are measured, the standards are 14 percent higher.

314–317. The answers are: 314-C, 315-E, 316-A, 317-D. *(Monif, pp 73, 197–198, 306, 455.)* Group A β-hemolytic streptococci can cause puerperal or postoperative pelvic infection. Outbreaks of puerperal fever are still reported on obstetrical services, though not at anywhere near the frequency of 50 years ago. When the disease does occur, a point source among the hospital personnel should be suspected.

Group B β-hemolytic streptococci, which also can cause puerperal fever, have recently been recognized as a major cause of severe neonatal infection. The organism can be isolated from the cervices of about 5 percent of all pregnant women; infection of the infant, which can result in sepsis, occurs as the infant passes through the vagina.

Toxoplasma gondii, a protozoan parasite, is transmitted by flies from cat feces to human food. Thus, humans can become infected by consuming infected meat that is inadequately cooked or by coming in direct contact with feces of an infected cat. Acute toxoplasmosis in a pregnant woman may cause a fulminant fetal infection; infected neonates may be born with microcephaly, intracranial calcification, or other symptoms.

An effective attenuated-virus vaccine is available for immunization against rubella. However, its use is contraindicated for pregnant women and commonly is associated with development of arthralgia in adults.

318–322. The answers are: 318-D, 319-C, 320-C, 321-B, 322-E. *(Pritchard, ed 16. pp 495–498, 508–510, 529–530, 588–594.)* Placenta previa is characterized by defective vascularization of the decidua, secondary to either inflammatory or atrophic changes; in this uncommon condition, the placenta is implanted over or near the internal os. Abruptio placentae (placenta abruption), which is associated very closely with maternal hypertension, is the premature separation of the placenta from the uterus. The Arias-Stella phenomenon, which refers to certain changes of the glands and epithelium of the endometrium, frequently is associated with ectopic pregnancy; however, this phenomenon also can occur whenever a conceptus is blighted and may be seen in intrauterine as well as extrauterine pregnancies. Spontaneous abortions histologically are accompanied by distended placental villi, hemorrhage into the decidua basalis, and evidence of necrotic changes in the region surrounding the hemorrhage.

Diagnosis and Management of Disorders of Labor, Delivery, and Puerperium

DIRECTIONS: Each question below contains five suggested answers. Choose the **one best** response to each question.

323. All of the following maneuvers may be employed in the vaginal delivery of a breech infant EXCEPT

(A) Saxtorph-Pajot maneuver
(B) Pinard maneuver
(C) Bracht maneuver
(D) Mauriceau-Smellie-Veit maneuver
(E) Prague maneuver

324. Which of the following factors would NOT be expected to reduce the risk of vaginal delivery for a full-term breech infant?

(A) Experience of the individual performing the delivery
(B) A previous full-term vaginal delivery
(C) Estimated fetal weight below 4000 g
(D) An x-ray revealing flexion of the fetal head
(E) A normal labor curve

Questions 325–326

A woman develops endometritis after a cesarean section has been performed. She is treated with penicillin and gentamicin but fails to respond.

325. Which of the following bacteria is resistant to these antibiotics and is likely to be responsible for this woman's infection?

(A) *Proteus mirabilis*
(B) *Bacteroides fragilis*
(C) *Escherichia coli*
(D) Alpha streptococci
(E) Anaerobic streptococci

326. The treatment of choice for this woman's condition would be

(A) polymyxin
(B) ampicillin
(C) cephalothin
(D) vancomycin
(E) clindamycin

327. The fetal monitoring strip shown below demonstrates which of the following?

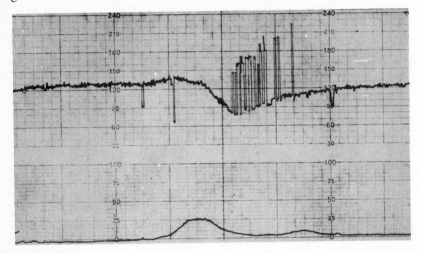

(A) A uteroplacental insufficiency pattern
(B) A cord pattern
(C) Head compression
(D) Uneventful labor
(E) Fetal death

---

328. Which of the following abnormal presentations is an absolute indication for a vertical cesarean section incision?

(A) Single footling breech at term
(B) Complete breech at 32 weeks
(C) Back up transverse lie
(D) Back down transverse lie
(E) Double footling breech at term

329. A 24-year-old primigravida is delivered vaginally after a long labor. Following delivery of the placenta, excessive bleeding from an atonic uterus is noted. Which of the following would NOT be an appropriate step in the management of this condition?

(A) Infusion of 20 units of oxytocin in a liter of normal saline over 30 minutes
(B) Intravenous injection of 5 units of oxytocin as a bolus
(C) Intramuscular injection of 0.2 mg methylergonovine
(D) Intrauterine lavage with a solution of prostaglandin F_{2x}
(E) Vigorous uterine massage

Questions 330–331

A 24-year-old primigravid woman, who is intent on breast-feeding, decides upon a home delivery. Immediately after the birth of a 4.1-kg (9-lb) infant, the patient bleeds massively due to extensive vaginal and cervical lacerations. She is brought in shock to the nearest hospital. Nine units of blood are transfused over 2 hours, and the blood pressure returns to a reasonable level. A hemoglobin value the next day is 7.5 g/100 ml, and 3 units of packed red blood cells are given.

330. The most likely late sequela to consider in this woman would be

(A) hemochromatosis
(B) Stein-Leventhal syndrome
(C) Sheehan syndrome
(D) Simmonds syndrome
(E) Cushing syndrome

331. Development of the sequela could be evident as early as

(A) 6 hours postpartum
(B) 1 week postpartum
(C) 1 month postpartum
(D) 6 months postpartum
(E) 1 year postpartum

332. The graph below depicts a labor curve for a woman, gravida 2, para 1, with intact membranes. This labor curve is compatible with which of the following conditions?

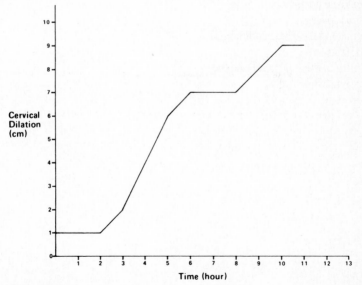

(A) Normal labor
(B) Protracted latent phase
(C) Protracted active phase
(D) Primary dysfunction
(E) Hypertonic dysfunction

333. Important techniques to prevent aspiration pneumonitis following obstetrical general anesthesia include all of the following EXCEPT

(A) fasting during labor
(B) antacid medications prior to anesthesia
(C) endotracheal intubation
(D) extubation with the patient in the lateral recumbent position with her head lowered
(E) extubation with the patient in the semierect position (semi-Fowler's)

334. Late deceleration patterns (type II dips) on a fetal monitoring strip represent

(A) cord compression
(B) pulmonary immaturity
(C) fetal hypoxia secondary to decreased perfusion of the intervillous spaces
(D) congenital cardiac conduction defects
(E) entry of the fetal head into the pelvic brim

335. Which of the following prerequisites for forceps deliveries does NOT apply to vacuum extraction deliveries?

(A) The head must be engaged
(B) The cervix must be completely dilated
(C) The position of the fetal head must be known
(D) The membranes must be ruptured
(E) None of the above

DIRECTIONS: Each question below contains four suggested answers of which **one or more** is correct. Choose the answer:

A	if	**1, 2, and 3**	are correct
B	if	**1 and 3**	are correct
C	if	**2 and 4**	are correct
D	if	**4**	is correct
E	if	**1, 2, 3, and 4**	are correct

336. Following a vaginal delivery, a woman develops a fever, lower abdominal pain, and uterine tenderness. She is alert, and her blood pressure and urine output are good. Large gram-positive rods suggestive of *Clostridia* are seen in a smear of the cervix. Management should include

(1) close observation for renal failure or hemolysis
(2) immediate radiographic examination for gas in the uterus
(3) high-dose antibiotic therapy
(4) hysterectomy

337. Barton forceps can be described by which of the following statements?

(1) It is useful when the fetal head is in a transverse position in a platypelloid pelvis
(2) It is useful when traction and rotation are to be performed simultaneously
(3) Application of the blades can be adjusted by a sliding lock
(4) The posterior blade is hinged

338. Hypertonic dysfunctional labor generally can be expected to

(1) cause little pain
(2) occur in the active phase of labor
(3) react favorably to oxytocin stimulation
(4) respond to sedation

339. Precipitate labor, which most often occurs in multiparous women, is associated with a greater-than-normal incidence of which of the following?

(1) Amniotic fluid embolism
(2) Fetal hypoxia
(3) Fetal cerebral trauma
(4) Cervical laceration

340. Predisposing factors to face presentation include

(1) contracted pelvis
(2) pendulous abdomen
(3) anencephalic fetus
(4) large fetus

341. A 25-year-old woman has recently delivered a 4-kg (8-1/2-lb) boy and is now experiencing heavy vaginal bleeding. The obstetrician should rule out which of the following causes of postpartum hemorrhage?

(1) Uterine atony
(2) Vaginal/cervical lacerations
(3) Retained placental fragments
(4) Blood dyscrasias

342. Fetal presenting positions that are usually undeliverable vaginally include

(1) brow
(2) mentum anterior
(3) mentum posterior
(4) left sacrum posterior

343. Chorioamnionitis develops in a woman whose membranes have ruptured at 35 weeks gestation; the fetus is alive. Management should include

(1) systemic antibiotics
(2) high-dose corticosteroids
(3) delivery by either a brief induction or cesarean section
(4) heparinization

344. A genital tract infection after delivery (puerperal infection) is characterized by which of the following statements?

(1) A temperature of 38°C (100.4°F) or higher on any 2 of the first 10 postpartum days (excluding the first day) is considered the standard definition of puerperal morbidity
(2) Iatrogenic causes are significant sources of infection
(3) The most common pathogens involved are those that normally inhabit the bowel and lower genital tract
(4) Anaerobic infections are common and frequently are caused by *Bacteroides*, *Peptostreptococcus*, or *Clostridium*

345. Agents that are currently approved in the United States by the Food and Drug Administration specifically for inhibition of premature labor include

(1) ethanol
(2) isoxsuprine
(3) terbutaline
(4) ritodrine

DIRECTIONS: The groups of questions below consist of lettered choices followed by several numbered items. For each numbered item select the **one** lettered choice with which it is **most** closely associated. Each lettered choice may be used once, more than once, or not at all.

Questions 346–349

For each clinical situation described below, choose the appropriate type of obstetrical forceps.

   (A) Simpson forceps
   (B) Kielland forceps
   (C) Barton forceps
   (D) Chamberlen forceps
   (E) Piper forceps

346. A breech delivery with an aftercoming head

347. The occiput transverse position in a flat pelvis

348. Fetal rotation

349. An elective low forceps delivery

Questions 350–352

For each of the following clinical descriptions, select the procedure that would be most appropriate.

   (A) External version
   (B) Internal version
   (C) Midforceps rotation
   (D) Low transverse cesarean section
   (E) Classic cesarean section

350. A 24-year-old primigravid woman, at term, has been in labor for 16 hours and has been 9 cm dilated for 3 hours. The fetal vertex is in the right occiput posterior position, at $+1$ station, and molded. There have been mild late decelerations for the last 30 minutes. Twenty minutes ago, the fetal scalp pH was 7.27; it is now 7.20

351. A 24-year-old woman (gravida 3, para 2) is at 40 weeks gestation. The fetus is in the transverse lie presentation

352. You have just delivered an infant weighing 2.5 kg (5.5 lb) at 39 weeks gestation. Because the uterus still feels large, you do a vaginal examination. A second set of membranes is bulging through a fully dilated cervix, and you feel a small part presenting in the sac. A fetal heart is auscultated at 60 beats per minute

Diagnosis and Management
of Disorders of Labor,
Delivery, and Puerperium
Answers

323. The answer is A. *(Pritchard, ed 16. pp 1070–1076.)* The Saxtorph-Pajot maneuver is the method by which axis traction is manually applied to an obstetrical forceps with a pelvic curve. The other maneuvers are all applicable to the vaginal delivery of a breech infant.

324. The answer is B. *(Pritchard, ed 16. pp 797–807.)* Vaginal delivery of the breech infant carries with it significant risks. These may be minimized through careful selection of patients, excluding those with large babies, abnormal labor patterns, and babies with hyperextended heads. The experience of the individual performing the delivery is directly proportional to its safety.

325. The answer is B. *(Monif, pp 8, 439–441.)* Infections caused by *Bacteroides fragilis,* a gram-negative anaerobic bacillus, are a significant obstetrical problem. Not only is the organism resistant to many commonly used antibiotics (including penicillin and gentamicin), but it is difficult to isolate, culture, and identify as well. The high incidence of gynecological and obstetrical *B. fragilis* infections may be due to the pathogen's predominance among the anaerobic bacteria of the lower bowel. Although the other organisms listed in the question also can cause postpartum infection, they are sensitive to antibiotic therapy with penicillin and gentamicin.

326. The answer is E. *(Monif, pp 8, 441–442.)* Clindamycin is the most effective antibiotic for treating women who have bacteroidosis. Chloramphenicol and tetracycline are alternative choices for antibiotic therapy in nonpregnant women; however, tetracycline-resistant strains of *Bacteroides fragilis* may be emerging. Lincomycin and erythromycin also can be effective in the management of affected women.

327. The answer is A. *(Lin, pp 319–327.)* The fetal monitoring strip that accompanies the question illustrates a uteroplacental insufficiency pattern. In this pattern, deceleration of the heart rate begins after the onset of the contraction, and the lowest rate occurs after the contraction has peaked. In addition there is a very slow return to the baseline. This is an ominous pattern and implies significant fetal hypoxia. Scalp pH sampling is warranted in this situation; and if acidosis is present and the pattern persists with subsequent contractions, rapid delivery should be performed. Diabetes mellitus and hypertensive states of pregnancy are diseases that typically compromise the functional capacity of the placenta.

328.   The answer is D. *(Pritchard, ed 16. pp 816–817.)* All of the listed abnormal presentations may, under various circumstances, be approached best via a vertical uterine incision. The back down transverse lie, however, requires a vertical incision since it allows neither the vertex nor the feet to gain proximity to a lower uterine transverse incision.

329.   The answer is B. *(Pritchard, ed 16. pp 426–429.)* Although oxytocin, prostaglandin, F_{2x}, and the ergot alkaloids are potent initiators of uterine contraction, vigorous uterine massage most often is an adequate first maneuver in the treatment of postpartum uterine atony. Although oxytocin is a safe, effective agent when administered as a dilute continuous infusion, several reports have shown it to cause hypotensive episodes when given as a concentrated bolus. In an actively bleeding patient, this effect must be avoided.

330–331.   The answers are: 330-C, 331-B. *(Pritchard, ed 16. pp 879–880.)* A disadvantage of home delivery is the lack of facilities to control postpartum hemorrhage. The woman described in the question delivered a large baby, suffered multiple soft-tissue injuries, and went into shock, needing 9 units of blood by the time she reached the hospital. Sheehan syndrome seems a likely possibility in this woman. This syndrome of anterior pituitary necrosis related to obstetrical hemorrhage can be diagnosed by 1 week postpartum, as lactation fails to commence normally. Although many modern women choose hormonal therapy to prevent lactation, the woman described in the question was intent on breast-feeding and so would not have received suppressant. She therefore could have been expected to begin lactation at the usual time. Other symptoms of Sheehan syndrome include amenorrhea, atrophy of the breasts, and loss of thyroid and adrenal function.

The other presented choices for late sequelae are rather far-fetched. Hemochromatosis would not be expected to occur in this healthy young woman, especially since she did not receive prolonged transfusions. Cushing, Simmonds, and Stein-Leventhal syndromes are not known to be related to postpartum hemorrhage.

It is important to note that home delivery is not a predisposing factor to postpartum hemorrhage.

332. The answer is C. *(Pritchard, ed 16. pp 385–387, 787–789.)* The labor described by the curve is characteristic of a protracted active phase. That the woman has entered the active phase is evident by the rate of dilatation (from 2 cm to 7 cm) over the space of 3 hours. The normal active phase progresses at a rate of at least 1.5 cm/h in a multiparous woman and 1.2 cm/h in a nulliparous woman. After 7 cm dilatation is reached in this patient, however, progress slows down to 2 cm over the next 4 hours, or 0.5 cm/h, and the active phase is said to be protracted. Another name for this condition is secondary arrest of labor. (Primary arrest of labor is arrest of progress before the active phase has begun.) If this woman's contractions are adequate by intrauterine monitoring and further progress does not occur, most obstetricians would perform a cesarean section. If hypotonic dysfunction were causing the protracted labor, some obstetricians would stimulate contractions with intravenous oxytocin.

333. The answer is E. *(Pritchard, ed 16. pp 440–441.)* Aspiration pneumonitis is the most common cause of anesthetic-related death in obstetrics. Its occurrence may be minimized by reducing both the volume and acidity of gastric contents, which is often difficult in the patient in labor whose stomach is extremely slow to empty. All obstetrical patients should be intubated for general anesthesia by a skilled individual. Extubation must be accomplished only after the patient is fully conscious and recumbent with her head turned to the side and lowered below the level of her chest.

334. The answer is C. *(Lin, p 319–327.)* Late deceleration patterns on a fetal monitoring strip result from fetal hypoxia caused by decreased perfusion, during contractions, of the intervillous spaces. A healthy fetus can tolerate the transient hypoxia resulting from contractions without exhibiting heart rate changes. Thus, late deceleration patterns are ominous, because they indicate that a fetus has very little reserve. Permanent damage of the central nervous system can result if the hypoxia is allowed to persist.

335. The answer is C. *(Pritchard, ed 16. pp 1045–1060.)* Vacuum extraction should be considered a form of forceps delivery in that it requires almost all of the same prerequisites as true forceps deliveries. The head must be engaged, membranes ruptured, and the cervix completely dilated. The only exception, and one of the few true advantages of vacuum extraction, is the lack of need to know the fetal position since proper application is irrespective of position.

336. The answer is A (1, 2, 3). *(Monif, pp 435–438.)* *Clostridia* can be seen in 5 to 10 percent of pelvic cultures. When the organism is found, appropriate antibiotic therapy (e.g., with penicillin) and close observation for gas gangrene, hemolysis, and renal failure are in order. Presumed identification on the basis of Gram stain alone or the presence of a mild infection without signs of sepsis or extrauterine involvement is not reason enough to proceed to hysterectomy.

337. The answer is B (1, 3). *(Pritchard, ed 16. p 1053.)* A special feature of Barton forceps is the hinged anterior blade. This type of forceps is useful when the fetal head is in a transverse position in a platypelloid pelvis; it should not be used, however, to perform simultaneous traction and rotation. Application of the forceps is by moving the hinged blade about the occiput or face; adjustment is made by a sliding lock.

338. The answer is D (4). *(Pritchard, ed 16. p 792.)* Hypertonic uterine dysfunction is characterized by a lack of coordination of uterine contractions, possibly caused by disorganization of the contraction gradient, which normally is greatest at the fundus and least at the cervix. This type of dysfunction usually appears during the latent phase of labor and is responsive to sedation, not oxytocin stimulation. The disorder is accompanied by a great deal of discomfort with little cervical dilatation (the familiar and painful false labor). After being sedated for a few hours, affected women usually awaken in active labor.

339. The answer is E (all). *(Pritchard, ed 16. pp 793–795.)* Precipitate labor is labor that either is extremely rapid or is not perceived by the patient or obstetrician. For example, some women who have had presacral neurectomy do not have painful contractions and thus may be unaware they are in labor. Rapid precipitate labor, which is more common, may be due to extremely strong or prolonged contractions. Because these contractions interfere with the proper oxygenation of fetal blood, fetal hypoxia can result. Extremely strong or long contractions coupled with an unyielding cervix or vagina may predispose to amniotic fluid embolism or tears of the cervix or vagina. Sudden delivery with rapid compression and decompression of the fetal head may cause cerebral trauma.

340. The answer is E (all). *(Pritchard, ed 16. pp 809–811.)* Face presentations occur in approximately 0.2 percent of deliveries. A large or anencephalic fetus, contracted pelvis, and pendulous abdomen all make extension of the head more likely. In addition, tumors of the anterior neck or multiple coils of umbilical cord around the neck may predispose to face presentation. Cesarean section commonly is necessary with face presentations; it may be avoided in many cases, however, if the decision is put off until the second stage of labor, when flexion or rotation to the mentum anterior position may occur.

341. The answer is E (all). *(Pritchard, ed 16. pp 878–879.)* Undoubtedly the most common cause of postpartum hemorrhage in the early puerperium is uterine atony, but vaginal lacerations and retained placental fragments must also be considered. Once these three major causes of hemorrhage have been ruled out, disorders of the coagulation system, either congenital (e.g., von Willebrand's disease) or acquired (e.g., disseminated intravascular coagulation), should be considered. The initial assessment of the woman described in the question should include a determination of previous bleeding problems, time since delivery, special problems encountered during delivery (e.g., manual removal of the placenta or vaginal laceration), quantity of blood loss, vital signs (including positional effect on blood pressure), and uterine consistency. Further diagnostic or therapeutic steps would depend upon this initial assessment of causative factors.

342. The answer is B (1, 3). *(Pritchard, ed 16. pp 812–813.)* In brow presentation, the fetal head is midway between flexion and extension. Except with an extremely small baby, engagement cannot occur unless flexion to vertex or extension to face presentation supervenes. In face presentation, delivery is by flexion rather than extension as in vertex presentations. Only the mentum anterior is capable of flexing under the pubic symphysis. The mentum posterior position does not allow flexion, because the neck is too short to go around the sacrum. The left sacrum posterior position is a variation of breech presentation. Although many present-day obstetricians would rarely deliver a breech vaginally, the breech presentation is by no means undeliverable.

343. The answer is B (1, 3). *(Monif, pp 297–299.)* The main mode of treatment for women who have chorioamnionitis is delivery. If the cervix is effaced and dilated, a brief induction could be undertaken; if the cervix is unripe, then abdominal delivery would be in order. Administration of potent antibiotics is important to prevent the development of sepsis in the mother. Although corticosteroids are not indicated in the treatment of women who have uncomplicated chorioamnionitis, such therapy might be valuable if septic shock develops. The use of steroids to accelerate pulmonary maturity would be inappropriate. Heparinization is not indicated in uncomplicated chorioamnionitis. Coagulation disorders, which may be a complication of severe infection, should not be treated unless there is uncontrollable bleeding.

344. The answer is E (all). *(Pritchard, ed 16. pp 893–904.)* The agents most responsible for puerperal infections are those normally found in the lower genital tract or in the bowel. These agents may be anaerobic bacteria (most commonly *Bacteroides, Peptostreptococcus,* and *Clostridium*) or aerobic bacteria (such as *Escherichia coli, Klebsiella, Pseudomonas,* and *Enterobacter*); infections caused by a combination of two or more pathogens occur frequently. Most puerperal infections are wound infections; trauma before or during delivery and iatrogenic bacterial contamination are significant etiological factors. Puerperal morbidity is defined as a temperature of 38°C (100.4°F) or higher occurring on any 2 of the first 10 postpartum days, excluding the first.

345. The answer is D (4). *(Barden, Obstet Gynecol 56:1–6, 1980.)* Although all the drugs listed in the question have been shown to successfully inhibit uterine activity, only ritodrine has been approved by the Food and Drug Administration for use in the treatment of preterm labor. This approval came in 1980 after world-wide experience with the drug had proven very favorable; in fact, ritodrine is expected to become the treatment of choice for premature labor in the next decade. Studies with ritodrine have shown it to be at least as useful as terbutaline or isoxsuprine with a minimum incidence of maternal hypotension noted. However, when using ritodrine, particularly if corticosteroids are administered concomitantly to accelerate fetal pulmonary maturity, care must be taken not to overload the patient with fluids and to be vigilant for early signs of pulmonary edema. This complication has been reported within the range of intake volumes that the healthy pregnant female could otherwise handle without difficulty. At present, the pathophysiology of this condition remains ill-defined.

346–349. The answers are: 346-E, 347-C, 348-B, 349-A. *(Pritchard, ed 16. pp 1041–1063, 1070–1075.)* Piper forceps were designed specifically for the delivery of the after-coming head in a vaginal breech delivery. They should never be applied until the head has fully entered the maternal pelvis and is engaged.

Barton forceps are designed for a transverse arrest in a platypelloid (flat) pelvis. The pelvic curve of the forceps is in an appropriate position vis-à-vis the maternal pelvis when the forceps are applied to the occiput transverse. Descent is then accomplished in this position, and rotation to the occiput anterior does not occur until the pelvic floor is reached. Rotation in the midplane thus is unnecessary; indeed, such rotation would be difficult in a flat pelvis.

Kielland forceps are designed specifically for rotation. They have very little pelvic curve and thus are unlikely to cause maternal soft-tissue injury during rotation. They can be used for occiput posterior or transverse positions, in which rotation is planned before traction is applied.

Simpson forceps are the prototype forceps for the molded head. They are useful for low forceps deliveries, and some obstetricians use Simpson or similar forceps for various rotation maneuvers.

Chamberlen forceps, the first true obstetrical forceps, were in use in the late sixteenth century.

350–352. The answers are: 350-D, 351-A, 352-B. *(Pritchard, ed 16. pp 645, 813–817, 1045–1046, 1081–1082, 1093–1095. Romney, ed 2. p 669.)* A woman who has been 9 cm dilated for 3 hours is experiencing a secondary arrest in labor. Deteriorating fetal condition (as evidenced, for example, by late decelerations and falling scalp pH) dictates immediate delivery. A forceps rotation would be inappropriate, because the cervix is not fully dilated. Cesarean section would be the safest and most expeditious method. Classic cesarean section is rarely used now because of greater blood loss and a higher incidence in subsequent pregnancies of rupture of the scar prior to labor. The best procedure would be a low transverse cesarean section.

A transverse lie is undeliverable vaginally. One treatment option is to do nothing and hope that the lie will be longitudinal by the time labor commences. The only other appropriate maneuver would be to perform an external cephalic version. This maneuver should be done in the hospital, with monitoring of the fetal heart. If the version is successful and the cervix is ripe, it might be best to take advantage of the favorable vertex position by rupturing the membranes at that point and inducing labor.

According to some studies, 25 percent of twins are diagnosed at the time of delivery. Although sonography or radiography can diagnose multiple gestation early in pregnancy, these methods are not used routinely in all medical centers. The second twin is probably the only remaining situation where internal version is permissible. Although some obstetricians might perform a cesarean section for a second twin presenting as a footling or shoulder, fetal bradycardia dictates that immediate delivery be done; and internal podalic version is the quickest procedure.

CLINICAL
GYNECOLOGY

Menstrual and Endocrine Disorders

DIRECTIONS: Each question below contains five suggested answers. Choose the **one best** response to each question.

353. Premenstrual staining is thought to be frequently associated with

(A) irregular shedding of the endometrium
(B) early corpus luteum failure
(C) anovulatory period
(D) hypothyroidism
(E) hyperthyroidism

354. In pituitary failure, the usual order of appearance of clinical deficiencies of the tropic hormones is

(A) somatotropin, thyrotropin, corticotropin, prolactin, gonadotropin
(B) thyrotropin, corticotropin, prolactin, gonadotropin, somatotropin
(C) corticotropin, prolactin, gonadotropin, somatotropin, thyrotropin
(D) prolactin, gonadotropin, somatotropin, thyrotropin, corticotropin
(E) gonadotropin, somatotropin, thyrotropin, corticotropin, prolactin

355. The presence of a uterus and fallopian tubes in an otherwise phenotypically normal male is due to

(A) lack of müllerian inhibiting factor
(B) lack of testosterone
(C) increased levels of estrogens
(D) 46,XX karyotype
(E) presence of ovarian tissue early in embryonic development

356. A 35-year-old woman presents with hypotension, cold intolerance, amenorrhea, waxy skin with multiple fine wrinkles, loss of axillary and pubic hair, and loss of skin pigmentation. Her urine sodium levels are normal. The most likely diagnosis is

(A) hypothyroidism
(B) Addison's disease
(C) panhypopituitarism
(D) malignant melanoma
(E) diabetes insipidus

357. In amenorrhea of hypopituitary origin one finds

(A) a normal FSH
(B) no withdrawal bleeding from progesterone alone
(C) no withdrawal bleeding from estrogen alone
(D) all of the above
(E) none of the above

358. The Sertoli-cell-only syndrome is characterized by which of the following levels of follicle-stimulating hormone (FSH), luteinizing hormone (LH), or both?

(A) Increased FSH levels
(B) Decreased FSH levels
(C) Increased LH levels
(D) Decreased LH levels
(E) Normal FSH and LH levels

359. In a 29-year-old woman taking oral contraceptives, amenorrhea is most likely due to

(A) pregnancy
(B) pituitary tumor
(C) Asherman syndrome
(D) relative progresterone excess in the contraceptive
(E) relative estrogen excess in the contraceptive

360. A 19-year-old man is seen because of late onset of puberty. The laboratory reports the man has azoospermia; and physical and historical findings indicate that he also has a poorly developed sense of smell. The most likely diagnosis is

(A) panhypopituitarism
(B) Reifenstein syndrome
(C) Klinefelter syndrome
(D) Kallman syndrome
(E) Turner syndrome

361. Increased incidences of endometrial hyperplasia and endometrial carcinoma have been described in patients with which of the following?

(1) Infertility
(2) Theca cell tumors of the ovary
(3) Polycystic ovaries
(4) Ingestion of conjugated estrogens

362. True statements regarding the empty-sella syndrome include which of the following?

(1) Headache is a common complaint
(2) Most affected patients have visual field defects
(3) It is most commonly seen in middle-aged, obese women
(4) X-ray of the sella turcica often reveals asymmetrical enlargement

DIRECTIONS: Each question below contains four suggested answers of which **one or more** is correct. Choose the answer:

A	if	**1, 2, and 3**	are correct
B	if	**1 and 3**	are correct
C	if	**2 and 4**	are correct
D	if	**4**	is correct
E	if	**1, 2, 3, and 4**	are correct

363. A 19-year-old woman consults you because of amenorrhea and galactorrhea of 1 year's duration. Her periods previously had been regular. She has had no other symptoms except for a mild headache. Diagnoses compatible with the findings on the CAT scan shown below include

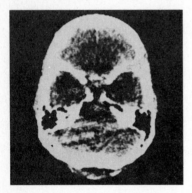

(1) empty-sella syndrome
(2) amenorrhea of a nonpituitary etiology
(3) microadenoma of the pituitary gland
(4) suprasellar lesion of a pituitary adenoma

364. Mammary-gland development is a common feature of patients who have

(1) testicular feminization
(2) Reifenstein syndrome
(3) Klinefelter syndrome
(4) Turner syndrome

365. Amenorrhea-galactorrhea is associated with

(1) hypothyroidism
(2) discontinuation of oral contraceptives
(3) abnormalities of the sella turcica
(4) the puerperium

366. Primary dysmenorrhea can be characterized by which of the following statements?

(1) Onset is usually with or shortly after menarche
(2) Pelvic examination is usually normal
(3) Irritability and depression are frequent emotional symptoms
(4) Symptoms are related to the release of prostaglandins in the menstrual fluid

367. True statements concerning anorexia nervosa include which of the following?

(1) It is seen predominantly in females, rarely in males
(2) Most affected patients have an obsessive-compulsive personality
(3) Mean 24-hour concentration of cortisol is twice normal
(4) Thyroid hormones are in the normal range

368. An 18-year-old woman has primary amenorrhea. Her growth and development have been normal. Work-up of this woman should include

(1) serum FSH and LH levels
(2) karyotype
(3) serum prolactin levels
(4) an endometrial biopsy

369. Asherman syndrome is characterized by which of the following?

(1) Biphasic basal body temperatures
(2) Diagnosis by endometrial biospy
(3) Amenorrhea
(4) Remission after removal of an intrauterine device

370. The causes of panhypopituitarism include

(1) postpartum hemorrhage
(2) Hand-Schuller-Christian disease
(3) temporal arteritis
(4) empty-sella syndrome

371. Signs or symptoms commonly associated wth anorexia nervosa but NOT with hypopituitarism include

(1) marked wasting
(2) loss of axillary and pubic hair
(3) elevated levels of human growth hormone
(4) decreased thyroid activity

372. Endometrial dysfunctional bleeding includes which of the following types?

(1) Estrogen breakthrough bleeding
(2) Estrogen withdrawal bleeding
(3) Progesterone breakthrough bleeding
(4) Progesterone withdrawal bleeding

DIRECTIONS: The groups of questions below consist of lettered choices followed by several numbered items. For each numbered item select the **one** lettered choice with which it is **most** closely associated. Each lettered choice may be used once, more than once, or not at all.

Questions 373–377

For each description that follows, select the type of sexual precocity with which it is most likely to be associated.

(A) True sexual precocity
(B) Incomplete sexual precocity
(C) Isosexual precocious pseudo-puberty
(D) Heterosexual precocious pseudopuberty
(E) Precocity due to gonadotropin-producing tumors

373. Defined by the presence of virilizing signs in girls

374. Characterized by the presence of premature adrenarche, pubarche, or thelarche

375. Can arise from cranial tumors or hypothyroidism

376. Stems from premature activation of the hypothalamus-pituitary system

377. Frequently caused by ovarian tumors

Questions 378–381

For each case history that follows, select the type of menstrual bleeding with which it most likely is associated.

(A) Progesterone breakthrough bleeding
(B) Progesterone withdrawal bleeding
(C) Estrogen breakthrough bleeding
(D) Estrogen withdrawal bleeding
(E) None of the above

378. A 24-year-old nulligravid woman is being evaluated for infertility. Her cycles are irregular, lasting from 30 to 90 days. Menstrual flow is usually heavy. She also has increasing hirsutism and obesity

379. A 55-year-old woman, 3 years postmenopause, is bothered by hot flashes. Her doctor orders conjugated estrogens (Premarin), 1.25 mg daily for 21 to 28 days. On the fourth month of Premarin therapy, the woman has heavy menstrual flow from the 25th to the 28th day

380. An 18-year-old woman complains of severe dysmenorrhea. She has regular periods every 28 days, with light flow on the first day, heavy flow on the second and third days, and light spotting on the fourth day

381. A 33-year-old woman is placed on one of the low-dose birth-control pills. Two weeks later, having taken nine of the birth-control pills, she has begun to have menstrual flow

Menstrual and
Endocrine Disorders

Answers

353. The answer is B. *(Kistner, ed 3. pp 625–626.)* The most common cause for premenstrual staining is an endocrine imbalance, usually considered an intrinsic, poorly understood corpus luteum failure. The endometrium shows varying degrees of progestational immaturity, and there may be disparity between glandular and stromal development. Treatment is often unnecessary.

354. The answer is E. *(Williams, ed 6. p 93.)* In pituitary failure, the tropic hormones usually disappear in the following order: gonadotropin, somatotropin, thyrotropin, corticotropin, and prolactin. When all the tropic hormones are gone, the diagnosis of pituitary failure is easy; however, in the evaluation of possible incipient pituitary failure, the sequential disappearance of these hormones can be an important diagnostic clue. Thus a woman who develops amenorrhea followed by symptoms of thyroid dysfunction should be suspected of having pituitary failure.

355. The answer is A. *(Speroff, ed 3. p 353.)* Individuals who appear to be normal males but who possess a uterus and tubes have an isolated failure of müllerian inhibiting factor. Their karyotype is 46,XY, testes are present, and testosterone production is normal.

356. The answer is C. *(Williams, ed 6. pp 92–97.)* The most likely diagnosis of the woman described in the question is panhypopituitarism. The associated hypotension results from a decrease in cortisone production, which is caused by a lack of corticotropin. Because the adrenal glands still maintain the ability to produce aldosterone, sodium levels are usually unchanged. Cold intolerance, amenorrhea, and changes in skin appearance and pigmentation are frequent signs of hypopituitarism. A patient who has hypothyroidism generally would present with different symptoms from those described, although cold intolerance may be encountered. A patient with Addison's disease would not be able to maintain body sodium. Malignant melanoma causes none of the presenting features described; and although diabetes insipidus may be a symptom of hypopituitarism, it does not cause the described symptomatology.

357. The answer is B. *(Speroff, ed 3. pp 148–154.)* With hypopituitary dysfunction one expects low gonadotropins and low circulating levels of endogenous estrogen. The progesterone challenge test will therefore be negative; however, the uterus will respond with bleeding to added estrogen administration.

358. The answer is A. *(Williams, ed 6. p 323.)* The Sertoli-cell-only syndrome is characterized by an increase in follicle-stimulating hormone (FSH) levels; luteinizing hormone (LH) levels remain normal. There are two major theories to explain how the testis controls FSH production. One is the "inhibin" theory, in which the germinal epithelium is thought to produce a water-soluble, nonsteroid substance that regulates FSH secretion. The other theory states that Sertoli cells secrete a steroid, possibly Δ^5-pregnenolone, that controls FSH production. In a testis containing only Sertoli cells, there would be no regulation on, hence no negative feedback of, FSH; therefore, FSH levels would be elevated.

359. The answer is D. *(Speroff, ed 3. pp 436–437.)* In all birth-control pill combinations the progestational effect dominates and produces a relatively shallow, atrophic endometrium that may be inadequate to yield withdrawal bleeding in some patients. This is reversible with resumption of normal ovarian function or estrogen supplementation.

360. The answer is D. *(Speroff, ed 3. pp 177, 380.)* The man described in the question has Kallman syndrome, which is a combination of hypogonadotropic eunuchoidism and hyposmia (an abnormally decreased sense of smell). Whether these two symptoms share a common etiology is not known. Panhypopituitarism and Reifenstein and Klinefelter syndromes all can lead to hypogonadism, but none are associated with abnormalities in the sense of smell. Turner syndrome is gonadal dysgenesis in an individual who has a 45,XO karyotype.

361. The answer is E (all). *(Kase, pp 860–861.)* Much evidence supports the relationship between unopposed estrogen and anovulation to hyperplasia of the endometrium. Any condition that increases endogenous estrogen levels, especially without regular progesterone challenges, may predispose the patient to uterine cancer.

362. The answer is B (1, 3). *(Speroff, ed 3. p 170. Yen, p 366.)* The empty-sella syndrome is a well-known condition in which an extension of the subarachnoid space is formed by the sella turcica. Pneumoencephalography, which will fill this space with air, is used as a diagnostic tool. Sella turcica x-ray usually reveals symmetrical enlargements. Individuals affected by this syndrome are frequently middle-aged women who are obese. The symptoms are generally nonspecific, with headaches being the most common complaint. The empty-sella syndrome is a benign condition that does not lead to pituitary failure. Inadvertent treatment for a pituitary tumor is probably the greatest hazard to the patient.

363. The answer is A (1, 2, 3). *(Speroff, ed 3. pp 153–156.)* The CAT scan that accompanies the question depicts a coronal section of the skull; the midline spherical area represents the sella turcica. In this study, the sella turcica is perfectly symmetric and normal in size. In the empty-sella syndrome, the sella is basically normal in configuration; a portion of arachnoid membrane herniates down through the diaphragm and compresses the active pituitary gland. Because microadenomas of the pituitary gland, which can produce prolactin and thus cause amenorrhea and galactorrhea, are usually less than 5 mm in size, they would not appear in the CAT scan shown. A suprasellar lesion of the pituitary gland would be larger than 5 mm and therefore would appear on most CAT scans.

364. The answer is A (1, 2, 3). *(Williams, ed 6. pp 449–460, 491–493.)* The degree of mammary-gland development depends on the relationship between estrogen and androgen production and utilization. Development of mammary tissue is significant in individuals who have testicular feminization, in which peripheral testosterone use is very low; Reifenstein syndrome, in which serum testosterone levels are reduced; or Klinefelter syndrome, in which testosterone production is decreased but estrogen production remains normal or near normal. On the other hand, mammary-gland development is not characteristic of Turner syndrome patients, who produce no androgen and very little estrogen.

365. The answer is E (all). *(Speroff, ed 3. pp 251–254.)* Amenorrhea and galactorrhea may be seen with all the listed clinical states. The differential diagnosis is difficult because of the multiple possible causes. For example, excessive estrogens such as with birth-control pills can reduce prolactin inhibiting factor (PIF), as can intensive suckling. Phenothiazine-derivative drugs are also known to have mammotrophic properties. Hypothryoidism appears to cause galactorrhea secondary to TRH stimulation of prolactin. With persistent elevated prolactin levels without obvious cause (e.g., breast-feeding) an evaluation for pituitary adenoma becomes necessary.

366. The answer is E (all). *(Romney, ed 2. pp 889–890.)* Primary dysmenorrhea is painful menstruation in the absence of pelvic disease that generally begins with the onset of regular ovulatory cycles. It is characterized by a combination of physical symptoms, such as pelvic cramps, nausea, vomiting, headache, and dizziness; and psychological symptoms, such as irritability, tension, and depression. Physical examination, including pelvic examination, is generally entirely normal. Recent investigations suggest that the symptomatology is caused by the local and systemic effects of prostaglandins released from menstrual fluid. Some investigators have reported an incidence of severe dysmenorrhea in 12 percent of women and moderate to severe dysmenorrhea in 45 percent of women. This frequency decreases with increasing parity.

367. The answer is A (1, 2, 3). *(Yen, pp 347–348.)* Anorexia nervosa is characterized by self-induced starvation and emaciation in the absence of organic disease. It is seen most commonly in adolescent girls and rarely occurs in boys. Most affected individuals have an obsessive-compulsive personality. It has been shown that the mean 24-hour cortisol concentration is twice normal because of increased circulation half-life and a decreased metabolic clearance rate. The daily cortisol production remains unchanged. These patients also have a low triiodothyronine (T_3) syndrome; both T_3 and thyroxine (T_4) are below normal values, with T_3 at a much lower level probably due to disturbance in the peripheral conversion of T_4 to T_3.

368. The answer is A (1, 2, 3). *(Speroff, ed 3. pp 145–149.)* In the workup of primary amenorrhea, serum FSH and LH determination can help to establish whether a woman has primary pituitary failure. A karyotype is important to rule out a genetic etiology, such as Turner syndrome. Determination of serum prolactin levels is now practicable and becoming more popular in the workup of amenorrhea. (Prolactin is elevated in many of the pituitary microadenomas causing amenorrhea.) An endometrial biopsy in the workup of primary amenorrhea is of no value whatsoever.

369. The answer is B (1, 3). *(Speroff, ed 3. p 156.)* Asherman syndrome is intrauterine synechia that usually follows a too-vigorous postpartum curettage. Affected women continue to ovulate, although they do not have menstrual bleeding; their basic body temperatures, therefore, are biphasic and normal. The diagnosis of Asherman syndrome is made by hysteroscopy or by hysterosalpingography. The etiology is not related to insertion of an intrauterine device (IUD), but IUDs have been utilized in treatment, because they separate the walls of the uterus after the adhesions are broken. However, a pediatric Foley catheter appears to be a better method of effecting the separation. After placement of the catheter, affected women should begin taking high doses of estrogen for 3 weeks a month, allowing the endometrium to regenerate.

370. The answer is E (all). *(Williams, ed 6. p 92–93.)* Postpartum panhypopituitarism is caused by hemorrhage in and subsequent necrosis of the pituitary gland, which is enlarged during pregnancy. Temporal arteritis and sickle cell anemia lead to panhypopituitarism by causing chronic vascular insufficiency of the pituitary gland. Hand-Schuller-Christian disease causes panhypopituitarism as a result of the infiltration of the gland by cholesterol-laden histiocytes. In the empty-sella syndrome, the pituitary gland becomes compressed within the sella. The pressure eventually necroses the tissue, and the gland becomes nonfunctional.

371. The answer is B (1, 3). *(Williams, ed 6. p 95.)* Patients who have anorexia nervosa, a loss of appetite due to emotional reasons, show a striking loss of body mass on physical examination; patients who have panhypopituitarism, however, show marked wasting only infrequently. Axillary and pubic hair are not lost in patients affected by anorexia nervosa, because circulating steroid levels are maintained. Steroid levels in panhypopituitarism, on the other hand, are low, causing loss of axillary and pubic hair. In panhypopituitarism, the human growth hormone level is extremely low and thyroid activity is decreased significantly; these values are either normal or elevated in anorectic individuals.

372. The answer is A (1, 2, 3). *(Speroff, ed 3. p 225.)* Estrogen withdrawal bleeding, estrogen breakthrough bleeding, and progesterone breakthrough bleeding are mechanisms of dysfunctional uterine bleeding, which is defined as bleeding that does not occur according to a normal cycle. Progesterone withdrawal bleeding is the mechanism by which normal menstrual flow commences. A woman normally ovulates on day 14, and the corpus luteum begins producing progesterone. When progesterone production ceases about 14 days later, menstruation ensues.

373–377. The answers are: 373-D, 374-B, 375-A, 376-A, 377-C. *(Speroff, ed 3. p 107. Williams, ed 6. pp 379–381, 632–636.)* True sexual precocity in girls is characterized by elevated gonadotropin levels and a normal ovulatory pattern. It represents premature activation of a normally operating hypothalamus-pituitary relationship. Although it usually is idiopathic, true sexual precocity can arise from cerebral causes as well as from hypothyroidism, polyostotic fibrous dysplasia, neurofibromatosis, and other disorders.

In girls who have precocious pseudopuberty, the endocrine glands, usually under neoplastic influences, produce elevated amounts of estrogens (isosexual precocious pseudopuberty) or androgens (heterosexual precocious pseudopuberty). Ovarian tumors appear to be the most common cause of isosexual precocious pseudopuberty; and some ovarian tumors, including dysgerminomas and choriocarcinomas, can produce so much gonadotropin that pregnancy tests are positive.

Incomplete sexual precocity, which usually is idiopathic, is characterized by only partial sexual maturity, such as premature thelarche, premature pubarche, or premature adrenarche. Incomplete sexual precocity can be accompanied by abnormal central-nervous-system function (e.g., mental deficiency).

In gonadotropin-producing tumors, high levels of gonadotropins, such as FSH, are produced with subsequent production of estrogen. Examples of these tumors are hepatoma, chorioepithelioma, and presacral tumors.

378–381. The answers are: 378-C, 379-D, 380-B, 381-A. *(Speroff, ed 3. pp 158–159.)* The four women described in the question represent the four different patterns of menstrual bleeding. The first woman is not ovulating, and because she is producing estrogen (in varying amounts) she continues to stimulate her endometrium; the endometrium grows to a point where it sloughs. This woman's bleeding thus is called estrogen breakthrough bleeding.

The second woman has estrogen withdrawal bleeding. She is producing very little estrogen or progesterone. Exogenous estrogen stimulates her endometrium to grow, but as soon as this stimulus is taken away the endometrium no longer has nutritive support and therefore is sloughed.

The third woman, who demonstrates progesterone withdrawal bleeding, represents a normally ovulating woman. At the end of 14 days, the corpus luteum stops producing progesterone and the endometrium loses is structural support and therefore is sloughed.

The fourth woman is taking birth-control pills and has a high progesterone-to-estrogen ratio. If the amount of progesterone is not high enough to support the endometrium in the early phases, and if structural support is poor, the endometrium will break down and the woman will have progesterone breakthrough bleeding.

Pelvic Relaxation, Infections, Endometriosis, and Infertility

DIRECTIONS: Each question below contains five suggested answers. Choose the **one best** response to each question.

382. The incidence of pelvic relaxational prolapse in parous women is approximately

(A) 10 percent
(B) 30 percent
(C) 50 percent
(D) 90 percent
(E) none of the above

383. Which of the following statements about pelvic tuberculosis is true?

(A) The primary site of involvement is the endometrium
(B) Infertility is a late complication
(C) The diagnosis can be made by endometrial biopsy
(D) The PPD skin test is positive in about half of affected women
(E) Treatment often restores fertility

384. An extremely anxious 50-year-old woman presents to your office and complains of soaking her underpants when arising in the morning. She also reveals that once initiated, she is unable to control micturition. The most likely diagnosis is

(A) detrusor dyssynergia
(B) short-urethra syndrome
(C) urgency incontinence
(D) urethral diverticulum
(E) overflow incontinence

385. Which is the most common sign of impending evisceration from a wound incision?

(A) Serous drainage
(B) Sanguineous drainage
(C) Serosanguineous drainage
(D) Abdominal pain with no drainage
(E) Abdominal contents in the wound

386. All of the following statements regarding gonorrhea are true EXCEPT that

(A) most women infected with *Neisseria gonorrhoeae* are asymptomatic
(B) the definitive diagnosis for gonorrhea depends upon a positive culture
(C) at diagnosis a seriologic test for syphilis should also be performed
(D) the usual reason for treatment failure is penicillin-resistant gonococci
(E) gonococcal infections resistant to both penicillin and spectinomycin should be treated with cefoxitin

387. The photomicrograph below shows a portion of uterine wall from a 43-year-old woman who has chronic pelvic pain and dysmenorrhea that is unresponsive to hormonal therapy. The most likely diagnosis is

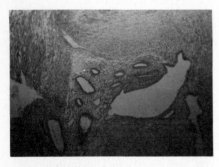

(A) endometriosis
(B) adenomyosis
(C) endometrial carcinoma
(D) ovarian carcinoma
(E) squamous cell carcinoma of the vulva

388. Conception rates are related to coital frequency. Which pattern is associated with the highest conception rate?

(A) Daily coitus throughout the cycle
(B) Alternate-day coitus throughout the cycle
(C) Single exposure at the presumed time of ovulation
(D) Alternate-day coitus around the presumed time of ovulation with abstinence during other parts of the cycle

389. A woman has been anuric for the first 48 hours after undergoing abdominal hysterectomy. Bilateral ligation of the ureters is suspected. Which of the following therapeutic measures should first be ordered?

(A) Observation only
(B) Ureteral catheterization
(C) Rapid dialysis
(D) Transabdominal deligation
(E) Bilateral nephrostomy

390. The most common site of endometriosis is the

(A) uterine surface
(B) anterior cul-de-sac
(C) uterosacral ligaments
(D) ovary
(E) rectovaginal septum

391. Varicoceles are related to male infertility. All of the following statements are true EXCEPT that

(A) varicoceles are found in approximately 15 percent of the general population
(B) the majority of varicoceles occur on the left side
(C) the size of the varix preoperatively correlates well with the prognosis of the success of surgery
(D) the most striking improvement with varicocele ligation is improvement in sperm motility
(E) the characteristic semen analysis associated with varicoceles shows the so-called stress pattern

392. An enterocele is best characterized by which of the following statements?

(A) It is not a true hernia
(B) It is a herniation of the bladder floor into the vagina
(C) It is a prolapse of the uterus and vaginal wall outside the body
(D) It is a protrusion of the pelvic peritoneal sac and vaginal wall into the vagina
(E) It is a herniation of the rectal and vaginal wall into the vagina

393. Asherman syndrome is associated with infertility. All of the following are true EXCEPT that

(A) symptoms include amenorrhea or hypomenorrhea
(B) patients are usually anovulatory
(C) diagnosis is made by hystero-salpingogram
(D) treatment consists of lysis of adhesions
(E) prophylactic antibiotics are a wise precaution for the surgical treatment of Asherman syndrome

394. All of the following statements about herpes genitalis are true EXCEPT that

(A) affected women may present with urinary retention
(B) many affected women have accompanying trichomoniasis or *Hemophilus vaginalis* vaginitis
(C) primary infections can be asymptomatic
(D) recurrent lesions tend to be disseminated and conspicuous
(E) use of tricyclic dyes can shorten the clinical course

395. The most common cause of genital prolapse is

(A) ascites
(B) chronic straining at bowel movements
(C) pregnancy
(D) menopause
(E) childbirth trauma

396. A 17-year-old girl comes to your office complaining of a foul-smelling vaginal discharge that is causing her a great deal of discomfort. On performing a speculum examination, a foamy, yellowish discharge is seen in the posterior fornix, and multiple petechiae are seen in the cervix. The most likely pathogen is

(A) *Candida albicans*
(B) *Trichomonas vaginalis*
(C) *Hemophilus vaginalis*
(D) *Hemophilus ducreyi*
(E) β-hemolytic streptococci

397. All of the following statements about vaginal candidiasis are true EXCEPT that

(A) monilial vulvovaginitis produces intense pruritis and burning
(B) the definitive diagnosis of infection depends upon isolating the responsible organism on Nickerson's culture medium
(C) examination of wet smears is a good substitute for culturing
(D) the organism may be visualized in a saline or KOH preparation
(E) the organism is a gram-positive, yeastlike fungus

398. All of the following statements about endometriosis are true EXCEPT that

(A) malignant changes are rare
(B) a diagnosis is established by history and physical examination
(C) it is more common in women in their reproductive years than in postmenopausal women
(D) affected women may present with infertility
(E) the most common site of involvement is the ovary

399. An 18-year-old woman comes to the emergency room with a complaint of vague lower abdominal pain for 1 week. Vital signs are stable except for a temperature of 37.8°C (100°F). Examination reveals tender adnexa bilaterally. Laparoscopy is performed and reveals bilateral hydrosalpinx. The next step in the management of this patient should be

(A) total abdominal hysterectomy and bilateral salpingectomy
(B) appropriate intravenous antibiotics
(C) bilateral salpingectomy
(D) posterior colpotomy
(E) further observation

400. All of the following steps are appropriate in the management of a woman who has a ruptured tubo-ovarian abscess EXCEPT

(A) preoperative antibiotic coverage consisting of penicillin and an aminoglycoside
(B) preoperative blood transfusion
(C) rapidly performed surgery (subtotal hysterectomy)
(D) bilateral salpingo-oophorectomy
(E) constant postoperative intestinal suction

401. All of the following statements about danazol are true EXCEPT that

(A) danazol is a progestational derivative of testosterone
(B) danazol will inhibit basal gonadotropin levels
(C) the endomentrial response to danazol is atrophy
(D) prompt return of menses and ovulation is noted when danazol is discontinued
(E) one should delay pregnancy at least 3 months after danazol therapy

DIRECTIONS: Each question below contains four suggested answers of which **one or more** is correct. Choose the answer:

A	if	**1, 2, and 3**	are correct
B	if	**1 and 3**	are correct
C	if	**2 and 4**	are correct
D	if	**4**	is correct
E	if	**1, 2, 3, and 4**	are correct

402. For couples in the United States between the ages of 18 and 28 years engaging in unprotected intercourse four times per week, which of the following conception rates are anticipated?

(1) Fifty percent will be pregnant by 4 months
(2) Sixty percent will be pregnant in 6 months
(3) Eighty percent will conceive in 1 year
(4) During the first year, the chance of conception per monthly cycle is 15 percent

403. If ureteral injury is recognized at the time of surgery, which of the following procedures could be recommended?

(1) A longitudinal slit should be made in the ureter below the injury and a polyethylene tube threaded into the bladder
(2) If the ureter is not severed, the site of injury should be drained intraperitoneally
(3) If the ureter is severed, ureteroureteral anastomosis should be attempted, regardless of the location of the injury
(4) If possible, the severed ureter should be implanted into the bladder

404. Luteal-phase defect is associated with faulty ovulation. Which of the following studies performed in the second half of the menstrual cycle would be helpful in making a diagnosis?

(1) Serum progesterone levels
(2) Urine pregnanetriol levels
(3) Endometrial biopsy
(4) Serum luteinizing hormome levels

405. There are several serologic tests for syphilis. True statements about nontreponemal tests and specific antitreponemal antibody tests include which of the following?

(1) The nontreponemal test should become positive within 7 to 14 days after chancre formation
(2) When successful treatment is employed early enough, the nontreponemal test will usually return to negative
(3) FTA is the most commonly used specific antititreponemal antibody test
(4) FTA remains positive indefinitely after treatment

406. During gynecological surgery, operative injuries to the ureter occur

(1) more frequently in association with vaginal rather than abdominal hysterectomy
(2) only rarely if periureteral tissue is dissected carefully
(3) most commonly when the ureter lies between the anterior vaginal wall and the base of the bladder
(4) often as a result of hasty reclamping of vessel clamps or ligatures

407. Histological features that are diagnostic for endometriosis include

(1) endometrial glands
(2) evidence of hemorrhage
(3) endometrial stroma
(4) decidual reaction in the surrounding tissue

---

408. The x-ray shown below reveals which of the following?

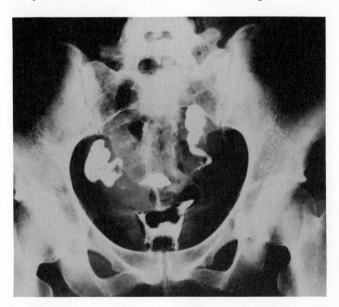

(1) Cornual obstruction
(2) Distended tubes
(3) Bilateral spill
(4) Bilateral hydrosalpinx

409. Retrograde menstruation is the most accepted explanation of the etiology of endometriosis. Which of the following statements may be cited as evidence for this theory?

(1) Inversion of the cervix of a monkey into the peritoneal cavity can cause endometriosis
(2) Endometrial tissue can be cultured successfully
(3) Menstrual blood can come from the ends of the fallopian tubes of some women
(4) Endometrial glands can arise from coelomic epithelium

410. Treatments commonly employed for women who have the vulvar lesion shown below include

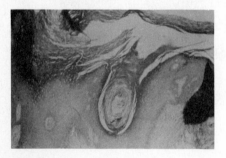

(1) podophyllum
(2) 5-fluorouracil
(3) cryosurgery
(4) simple vulvectomy

411. At the present time, treatment of women who have endometriosis can consist of single-agent therapy with

(1) androgens
(2) progestational agents
(3) nonsteroidal gonadotropin inhibitors
(4) estrogens

412. Which of the following conditions can predispose to vaginal infection with *Candida albicans*?

(1) Pregnancy
(2) Antibiotic therapy
(3) Adrenocorticosteroid therapy
(4) Presence of an intrauterine device

DIRECTIONS: The groups of questions below consist of lettered choices followed by several numbered items. For each numbered item select the **one** lettered choice with which it is **most** closely associated. Each lettered choice may be used once, more than once, or not at all.

Questions 413–416

Match each infertility test with the appropriate time for it to be done in a 28-day cycle.

(A) day 8
(B) day 14
(C) day 24
(D) day 2

413. Hysterosalpingography

414. Postcoital testing

415. Endometrial biopsy

416. Serum progesterone

Questions 417–420

For each clinical presentation that follows, select the antibiotic with which it should be treated.

(A) Gentamicin
(B) Ampicillin
(C) Tetracycline
(D) Cephalothin
(E) A sulfonamide antibiotic

417. A 23-year-old woman who has had a septic abortion has positive blood cultures with an organism that is identified as an aerobic gram-negative rod

418. A 28-year-old woman who is in her thirty-seventh week of pregnancy develops a urinary tract infection with *Escherichia coli*

419. A 34-year-old single woman develops a *Mycoplasma hominis* infection

420. A 28-year-old woman at 4 weeks gestation develops asymptomatic bacteriuria

Questions 421–424

For each description that follows, select the operative procedure with which it is most likely to be associated.

(A) Salpingoplasty
(B) Salpingostomy
(C) Salpingolysis
(D) Fimbriolysis
(E) Uterotubal implantation

421. Forming a patent entry site in the fundal portion of the uterus and attaching the oviduct

422. Section of adhesions causing conglutination of the distal end of the oviduct

423. Cutting adhesions around the uterine tube

424. Opening up a previously formed hydrosalpinx

Questions 425–428

For each clinical description that follows, select the appropriate disorder.

(A) Neurogenic bladder
(B) Overflow incontinence
(C) Stress incontinence
(D) Vesicovaginal fistula
(E) Urgency incontinence

425. A 45-year-old woman states that she has had increasing difficulty holding urine after feeling the need to void. She occasionally loses urine when sitting down

426. A 43-year-old woman, who recently underwent an anterior vaginal repair, complains of constant perineal wetness and loss of urine while standing. She does not feel the urge to void

427. A 28-year-old diabetic woman reports that she loses large volumes of urine without warning. She says that she can overcome the problem by frequent, voluntary emptying of the bladder

428. A 26-year-old woman, who has four children, is worried because her daily jogging seems to be causing urinary dribbling

Questions 429–433

Match the following.

(A) *Candida albicans*
(B) *Trichomonas vaginalis*
(C) *Neisseria gonorrhoeae*
(D) *Corynebacterium vaginale (Hemophilus vaginalis)*
(E) Atrophic (senile) vaginitis

429. A frequent cause of nonspecific vaginitis

430. Diabetes mellitus may be a predisposing factor

431. Typically produces a frothy discharge

432. Typically produces a grossly recognizable, punctate hemorrhagic vaginal mucosa ("strawberry spots")

433. Treatment with an estrogen cream may be effective

Pelvic Relaxation, Infections, Endometriosis, and Infertility

Answers

382. The answer is C. *(Kase, p 677.)* Pelvic relaxation is very common in parous women; however, the relaxation is not always symptomatic enough to warrant operative correction. Indications for surgical correction are directly related to patient discomfort during intercourse and the development of urinary symptoms.

383. The answer is C. *(Green, ed 3. pp 270–272.)* Pelvic tuberculosis is usually secondary to tuberculous infection in another part of the body, most often the lung. It is thought that the infection spreads hematogenously from the fallopian tubes, the primary site of pelvic infection, into the endometrial cavity. Although the endometrium is only secondarily affected, endometrial biopsy often is the easiest method of diagnosis. The tuberculin skin (PPD) test usually is positive. Affected women most often present with pelvic pain, dysmenorrhea, dysparenua, irregular menses, and cervical lesions. In view of primary tubal involvement, infertility is an early manifestation; and even with proper treatment, affected women have only a poor chance of regaining their childbearing capacity.

384. The answer is A. *(Green, ed 3. pp 552–556.)* True urinary stress incontinence results from a deficiency of the normal anatomical support of the bladder neck and urethra. The condition that most often mimics true urinary stress incontinence is detrusor dyssynergia, which in the majority of cases has a psychosomatic origin and often produces a "voiding" type of leakage associated with a change in position, such as arising from bed in the morning. The short-urethra syndrome results in continuous leakage of urine regardless of position or stress, and pure urgency incontinence, which is often secondary to a nonbacterial trigonitis or cystitis, often results in sudden, uncontrollable micturition. Urethral diverticula are not associated with incontinence. Overflow incontinence would be suggested by frequent voiding of small amounts of urine with a significant residual urine volume noted on catheterization.

385. The answer is C. *(Mattingly, ed 5. pp 176–179.)* Serosanguineous drainage occurs very frequently before evisceration from the incision. Drainage can be accompanied by pain or by the feeling that something is "giving way." Serous or sanguineous drainage often is noted postoperatively and usually suggests involvement of the superficial wound.

386. The answer is D. *(Kase, p 604.)* Gonococcus can persist asymptomatically in women for weeks to months. Although gonorrhea may be suspected clinically, a positive culture should be obtained before informing the patient that she is infected. There is an increased incidence of syphilis in women with gonorrhea, and such should be evaluated. The usual reason for treatment failure is reinfection; therefore, it should be stressed that both partners should be treated. Cefoxitin is the treatment of choice for gonorrhea resistant to penicillin and spectinomycin.

387. The answer is B. *(Novak, ed 8. pp 280–290.)* The histological and historical evidence presented in the question suggests adenomyosis. Adneomyosis is defined as endometrial tissue outside of the endometrial cavity and confined to the uterine wall. Tufts of endometrial tissue can be surrounded by areas of smooth muscle (myometrium), as in the accompanying photomicrograph. Endometriosis is defined as endometrial tissue outside of the uterus. Because the lesion shown is certainly benign, ovarian carcinoma and carcinoma of the vulva are ruled out. Women who have adenomyosis suffer from chronic pelvic pain and dysmenorrhea, usually associated with an enlarged uterus. A diagnosis is rarely made clinically and usually depends on pathological examination.

388. The answer is A. *(Kase, p 426.)* Barrett and Marshall found that daily coitus was associated with a 68 percent chance of pregnancy and alternate-day intercourse with a 43 percent chance. A single episode of intercourse around ovulation carries only a 30 percent chance of impregnation.

389. The answer is B. *(Mattingly, ed 5. pp 299–300.)* Bilateral ureteral obstruction, if unrecognized or unrelieved, can cause death in 7 to 10 days. Once the presence of bilateral ureteral obstruction is suspected, bilateral ureteral catheters should be passed in order to demonstrate and, if possible, overcome the obstructions. If obstruction persists, bilateral nephrostomy should be performed; if, 6 to 8 weeks later, the obstructions still cannot be overcome, ureteral surgery should be undertaken.

390. The answer is D. *(Kase, p 478. Romney, ed 2. p 933.)* The most common site of endometriosis is the ovary. Superficial serosal lesions also are common, especially on the uterine and tubal surfaces and in scattered locations on the pelvic serosa. Endometrial implants may also be found on the uterosacaral ligaments, round ligaments, in the rectovaginal septum, on the pelvic peritoneum covering the uterus, tubes, rectum, sigmoid, or bladder, at the umbilicus, in laparotomy scars, hernial sacs, the appendix, vagina, vulva, cervix, tubal stumps, or lymph nodes.

391. The answer is C. *(Kase, pp 438–439.)* The incidence of varicoceles in the general population is about 15 percent, but 40 percent of males with infertility are found to have varicoceles. Because of the anatomy and physiology, varicoceles are more likely to occur on the left side. There is no correlation between the size of the varix with fertility prognosis. The characteristic "stress pattern" seen with varicoceles is decreased number of sperm, decreased motility, and increased abnormal forms.

392. The answer is D. *(Mattingly, ed 5. pp 603–607.)* An enterocele is the protrusion of the pelvic peritoneal sac and the vaginal wall into the vagina. It is a true hernia, and it may be either congenital or associated with a uterine prolapse. Enteroceles can also occur following vaginal hysterectomy if the cul-de-sac is not adequately obliterated. Most commonly, patients with enteroceles complain of a mass protruding from the vagina when they strain, cough, sneeze, or perform other activities associated with the Valsalva maneuver—that is, activities causing pressure (by exhalation) against a closed glottis. Also, if intestines are present in the herniated sac, local discomfort will probably result.

393. The answer is B. *(Kase, p 457.)* Ovulation is not affected in Asherman syndrome. Because of the decreased amount of functional endometrium, hypomenorrhea or amenorrhea are common. The best diagnostic study is the hysterosalpingogram under fluoroscopy. Hysteroscopy with lysis of adhesions is the treatment of choice. Prophylactic antibiotics may improve success rates.

394. The answer is D. *(Romney, ed 2. pp 924–925.)* The symptoms of primary herpes genitalis, which include blisters, ulcers, pain, and urinary retention, are often severe and may persist for several weeks. Several studies have shown that a number of women who show no signs of herpes genitalis have antibodies to herpes simplex virus type 2, the causative agent of the disease; this finding indicates that these women have had previous, asymptomatic infections. Recurrent infections, which occur commonly, are localized and often hard to identify. Treatment of herpetic lesions is being attempted with many agents. The most promising of those already approved by the FDA is acycloguanosine (Acyclovir). Many newer agents are still under investigation.

395. The answer is C. *(Kase, p 680.)* Although all these conditions may lead to genital prolapse, it is believed that pregnancy per se is the most important. Increased cortisol and progesterone production during pregnancy may "soften" the fascial supports of the uterus and vagina. In addition, the weight of the pregnant uterus is an important factor in initiating genital prolapse during pregnancy.

396. The answer is B. *(Green, ed 3. p 277. Parsons, ed 2. pp 766, 771.)* Foamy, foul discharge accompanied by cervical petechiae, which are often described as "strawberrylike" in appearance, confirms the diagnosis of trichomoniasis. The latter finding is not seen in any other form of vaginitis. In candidiasis, the discharge is less abundant, and on speculum examination, thick, cheeselike plaques can be seen clinging to the vaginal mucosa. Infection with *Hemophilus vaginalis* produces a grayish, malodorus discharge and does not cause as much intense itching and burning as the previous two pathogens described. *Hemophilus ducreyi* is the causative organism of chancroid (soft chancre).

397. The answer is C. *(Kase, pp 596–597.)* Examination of a wet smear may be misleading because 30 percent of patients with vaginitis with a negative wet smear are found to have a positive culture for *Monilia.* Although definitive diagnosis of infection rests with isolating the organism using an appropriate culture medium, a positive diagnosis can often be made by microscopic examination of vaginal secretions, thus obviating the need for performing a culture. On the other hand, examination of wet smears is not a substitute for culture. In all cases in which wet smear examination proves negative, a culture must be used to rule out *C. albicans* as a cause of inflammation.

398. The answer is B. *(Romney, ed 2. pp 932–933, 938–940.)* Endometriosis, which most commonly involves the ovaries, is a disease of women in their reproductive years, especially between the ages of 30 and 40 years. The disease is usually benign. The definitive diagnosis of endometriosis rarely can be established short of surgery or diagnostic laparoscopy. Diagnosis is aided by the presence of vulvar, vaginal, or cervical lesions, which can be biopsied; palpable cul-de-sac nodules; and a history of dysmenorrhea and infertility.

399. The answer is B. *(Mattingly, ed 5. pp 259–264.)* In the initial management of an acute pelvic infection, the use of surgery is rarely indicated. Laparoscopy is a useful tool for providing a definitive diagnosis and indicating the extent of the disease. In most cases of acute pelvic infection, 24 to 72 hours of appropriate intravenous antibiotic therapy followed by 1 week of oral therapy will produce a positive response. Definitive surgery can be recommended for the older patient whose childbearing functions have been fulfilled. Posterior colpotomy is performed for the purpose of establishing drainage, when the abscess is fluctuant and located in the midline.

400. The answer is A. *(Mattingly, ed 5. pp 269–271.)* An important aspect that is often overlooked in the management of a woman who has a tubo-ovarian abscess is preoperative antibiotic coverage for *Bacteroides fragilis.* Because penicillin combined with an aminoglycoside can cover all potential pathogens except *B. fragilis,* clindamycin, carbenicillin, or chloramphenicol should be added to the antibiotic regimen. Because patients are put in Trendelenberg position, rapid surgery is required; thus, a subtotal hysterectomy frequently is performed. For most patients, bilateral salpingo-oophorectomy also is indicated, and postoperative intestinal suction is recommended.

401. The answer is B. *(Kase, p 480.)* Danazol is a progestational compound derived from testosterone. It induces a pseudomenopause but does not alter basal gonadotropin levels. It appears to act as an antiestrogen and will cause endomentrial atrophy. Cyclic menses return almost immediately upon danazol withdrawal. It is felt that the endometrium is poorly developed with danazol use and that three menstrual cycles should be allowed to go by before conceiving so as to avoid a higher risk of spontaneous abortion and other poor implantation problems.

402. The answer is E (all). *(Kase, p 426.)* These figures are used when investigating a couple for potential fertility. Approximately 20 percent of couples attempting pregnancy for 1 year will be unsuccessful. Half of those will spontaneously conceive during the second year. Half of those remaining, or approximately 5 percent, will benefit from specific therapy.

403. The answer is D (4). *(Mattingly, ed 5. pp 300–306.)* Following an injury to the ureter during surgery, a drain should be placed extraperitoneally. If a polyethylene catheter is inserted, it should be placed above the site of injury so that urine is drained before arrival at the site of injury. Ureteroureteral anastomosis should be done only if reimplantation into the bladder is not feasible. Implanting a severed ureter into the bladder is the procedure of choice.

404. The answer is B (1, 3). *(Speroff, ed 3. pp 478–482.)* A short luteal phase is defined as ovulation with poor production of progesterone in the second half of the cycle. Progesterone levels at that time of less than 7 ng/ml are diagnostic. Endometrial biopsy also is crucial to the diagnosis of this defect, because the endometrium will be out of phase with the time of cycle. For example, a biopsy taken on day 26 of the cycle will resemble endometrium of day 24 because of decreased progesterone stimulation. Pregnanetriol is a breakdown product of 17-hydroxyprogesterone, and levels are not helpful in diagnosing this condition. Determination of the level of pregnanediol, which is a metabolic product of progesterone excreted in the urine, is a helpful test. Serum luteinizing hormone levels have no correlation with the presence of a luteal-phase defect.

405. The answer is E (all). *(Kase, p 605.)* Current nontreponemal tests include RPR and VDRL. These tests are useful for screening. They become positive 1 to 2 weeks after chancre formation and remain positive indefinitely if untreated. The fluorescent treponemal antibody absorbtion test (FTA-ABS) is the most commonly used antitreponemal test. FTA does become positive earlier than RPR and will remain positive indefinitely even after treatment. One cannot follow FTA titers as a measure of cure or reinfection.

406. The answer is D (4). *(Mattingly, ed 5. pp 293–295.)* Operative injuries to the ureter are associated more commonly with abdominal hysterectomy than vaginal hysterectomy. The most common site of injury occurs near the region of the uterine vessels. Because the blood supply to the ureter arises from the periureteral tissue, dissection should be avoided; even careful dissection results in a significant percentage of ureteral injuries, and the incidence of fistula formation is increased if the blood supply is compromised. Slippage of vessels from clamps or ligatures can lead to ureteral injury if the vessels are reclamped hastily in an effort to stop the resultant bleeding.

407. The answer is A (1, 2, 3). *(Green, ed 3. p 334.)* In view of the importance of accuracy in diagnosing endometriosis, strict, definitive criteria must be used. The triad of histological findings that is diagnostic for endometriosis consists of the presence of endometrial glands and endometrial stroma and evidence of recent or old hemorrhage. In women who are pregnant or who are receiving certain forms of hormonal therapy, a significant decidual reaction may be seen; this feature, however, is by no means diagnostic for endometriosis.

408. The answer is C. (2, 4). *(Kistner, ed 3. pp 290–295.)* The x-ray presented reveals bilateral hydrosalpinx and distended tubes; no spill is noted at the fimbriated extremity. These findings are suggestive of chronic pelvic inflammatory disease. Both cornual areas appear normal, and there is no spill into the peritoneal cavity.

409. The answer is A (1, 2, 3). *(Speroff, ed 3. p 494.)* Retrograde menstruation is currently believed to be a major cause of endometriosis. Supporting this belief are the following findings: inversion of the uterine cervix into the peritoneal cavity can cause the monkey to develop endometriosis; endometrial tissue is viable outside the uterus; and blood can issue from the ends of the fallopian tubes of some women during menstruation. The fact that endometrial implants can occur in the lung implies that lymphatic or vascular routes of spread of the disease also are possible. Another theory of the etiology of endometriosis entails the conversion of coelomic epithelium into glands resembling those of the endometrium.

410. The answer is B (1, 3). *(Novak, ed 8. pp 28–30.)* The lesion shown in the figure accompanying the question is condyloma acuminatum, also known as a venereal wart; it is a squamous lesion caused by the papilloma virus. The lesion reveals a treelike growth microscopically, with a mantle that shows marked ancathosis and parakeratosis. Occasionally hyperkaratosis is noted. The treatment is local excision, cryosurgery, or podophyllum, which is a locally acting, mild antimetabolite. 5-Fluorouracil is a very potent antimetabolite, and simple vulvectomy is too expensive and radical a surgical procedure for removal of this benign, self-limiting lesion.

411. The answer is A (1, 2, 3). *(Green, ed 3. pp 342–344.)* The major hormonal agents used at this time in the treatment of women who have endometriosis are progestins and androgens. Hormonal therapy has proved especially useful for women whose symptoms are mild. Because pregnancy can lessen the severity of endometriosis, estrogen therapy was tried as a possible treatment; the incidence of side effects and complications proved to be quite high, however, and estrogens now are used only for treatment of women with breakthrough-type bleeding. Gonadotropin inhibition is now possible without the use of steroid therapy.

412. The answer is A (1, 2, 3). *(Monif, pp 242–243.)* Pregnancy is associated with an increase in the incidence of monilial infections, probably because of an increase in glycogen content in the vaginal mucosa. Antibiotic therapy clearly increases the likelihood of candidiasis (moniliasis), perhaps because it eliminates susceptible bacteria that compete with *Candida* for available nutrients. Steroid therapy may involve inhibition of catabolic-enzyme release. No association exists between the use of intrauterine devices and a predisposition toward monilial infections.

413–416. The answers are: 413-A, 414-B, 415-C, 416-C. *(Kase, pp 429–430.)* Hysterosalpingography should be performed sufficiently after menses to avoid retrograde movement of menstrual fluid through the tubes and sufficiently before ovulation so as not to interfere with possible conception or implantation. Postcoital testing is best done around ovulation to take advantage of optimal cervical mucus. Endometrial biopsy and serum progesterone are used to document ovulation and are best done between days 24 and 26 of the cycle.

417–420. The answers are: 417-A, 418-B, 419-C, 420-E. *(Monif, pp 9, 26, 159. Romney, ed 2. p 725. Willson, pp 37, 426.)* Gentamicin, an aminoglycoside similar to kanamycin and streptomycin, is not absorbed after oral administration. It is the drug of choice for women who have severe infections caused by gram-negative aerobes.

The penicillins are nontoxic for pregnant women. Ampicillin is used effectively for treating urinary tract infections and acute pyelonephritis. Ampicillin can cause a decrease in the urinary excretion of estriol in pregnancy. The exact reason for this is unclear.

Although *Mycoplasma hominis* commonly is found in the genital tract, its role in producing infections is unclear. Documented mycoplasmal infections are best treated with tetracycline, unless the affected woman is pregnant, as tetracycline deposition in fetuses can cause abnormal growth and permanent mottling of the teeth. Also, large doses of the drug may cause hepatic degeneration in the mother.

Pregnant women with asymptomatic bacteriuria can be treated effectively and safely with sulfonamides up until the last months of pregnancy—after which sulfonamides are contraindicated. In late pregnancy, this antibiotic crosses the placenta and competes with bilirubin for binding sites in the fetus, which can lead to hyperbilirubinemia and kernicterus in the neonate.

421–424. The answers are: 421-E, 422-D, 423-C, 424-B. *(Sciarra, ed 2, vol 1, chap 74, pp 1–18.)* Salpingolysis, salpingoplasty, and uterotubal implantation are the major surgical techniques utilized by tubal surgeons. A salpingolysis is merely the cutting of adhesions surrounding the fallopian tube. Salpingoplasty, which is performed on the fimbriated end of the tube, is divided into two parts: fimbriolysis, which is a simple cutting of adhesions causing the fimbria to conglutinate in the midline, and salpingostomy, which is creation of an opening in tubes that were completely closed with hydrosalpinx, usually secondary to infection. On occasion, the tube is occluded at the cornual area, which must be excised, and a new opening into the uterus must be created; this procedure is uterotubal implantation. These procedures are commonly use to correct infertility problems related to lack of tubal patency or mobility interfering with ovum pickup/transport. Predisposing factors include endometriosis, pelvic inflammatory disease, appendicitis, and prior tubal ligation.

425–428. The answers are: 425-E, 426-D, 427-A, 428-C. *(Romney, ed 2. pp 958–962.)* Urgency incontinence resulting from hyperactivity of the detrusor muscle is associated with the loss of large amounts of urine just after a woman has had an urge to void. Sudden motions can trigger the urge.

Small fistulas can result from improperly performed surgery that has created an unnoticed entry into the bladder. Affected patients, when recumbent, will pool urine in the vagina.

Diabetes as well as neurological disorders can be associated with neurogenic bladder. Reflex emptying, which usually is spasmodic and not accompanied by a sensation of a full bladder, is characteristic of the disorder.

Characteristically, stress incontinence is the loss of urine caused by sudden increases in intraabdominal pressure. The condition is uncommon in women who never have been pregnant.

Conditions that cause pressure on or constriction of the bladder neck can lead to an overdistended bladder. Overflow incontinence also occurs not infrequently among elderly patients.

429–433. The answers are: 429-D, 430-A, 431-B, 432-B, 433-E. *(Sciarra, ed 2, vol 1, chap 24, pp 8–9; chap 26, pp 1–6.)* Many cases of nonspecific vaginitis are caused by *Corynebacterium vaginale*. These women usually complain of a characteristic malodorous, grayish vaginal discharge. On wet mounts, the diagnosis is made by visualizing the "clue cells," which are epithelial cells with large numbers of adherent coccobacilli. The recommended treatment is ampicillin, although vaginal sulfa creams are also effective.

Besides diabetes mellitus, other predisposing factors of candidiasis include pregnancy, the use of antibiotics, immunosuppressive medications, and possibly oral contraceptives. Affected individuals usually complain of severe pruritus and thick, cheeselike vaginal discharge. Wet mounts show chracteristic yeast cells and hyphae. The primary mode of treatment is the vaginal application of an antifungal agent, such as nystatin.

Trichomonas vaginalis classically gives rise to a yellowish, frothy discharge, which is foul smelling and causes pruritus. The pathognomonic "strawberry spots," which consist of punctate hemorrhagic spots on the vaginal mucosa, can sometimes be seen. The diagnosis is made by observing the characteristic motile protozoan on wet mounts. The mainstay of treatment is oral metronidazole, either in a single dose of 2 g or 250 mg three times a day for 7 to 10 days. Metronidazole has a disulfiramlike effect, and women taking it should refrain from consumption of alcohol. Vaginal suppositories of clotrimazole, 100 mg once a day for 7 days, are also effective and are preferred by some because of carcinogenicity found in rodents treated with metronidazole.

Postmenopausal women who present with symptoms like itching, irritation secondary to dryness, and dyspareunia often have atrophic (senile) vaginitis. Due to the lack of estrogen, the vaginal mucosa becomes very thin and easily irritable. This condition responds well to either oral intake of estrogen or local application of estrogen creams.

The Bartholin's glands, endocervical glands, and fallopian tubes can all be infected by *Neisseria gonorrhoeae,* but an infection of the vaginal mucosa is uncommon.

Benign and Malignant Neoplasms

DIRECTIONS: Each question below contains five suggested answers. Choose the **one best** response to each question.

434. Which of the following statements is characteristic of endometrioid carcinoma of the ovary?

(A) It accounts for the majority of epithelial ovarian carcinomas
(B) It is distinguishable from adenocarcinoma of endometrial origin
(C) Squamous differentiation is uncommon
(D) Concomitant adenocarcinoma of the endometrium can occur
(E) Approximately 80 percent of endometrioid ovarian carcinomas are accompanied by ovarian endometriosis

435. In stage II carcinoma of the endometrium

(A) the length of the uterine cavity is less than 8 cm
(B) the corpus and the cervix are involved
(C) there is extension to involve the parametrium
(D) there is extension to the ovaries
(E) there is metastasis to the bladder

436. The primary mode of treatment for endometrial carcinoma confined to the uterine corpus is

(A) external beam radiation
(B) intracavitary radium
(C) hysterectomy
(D) chemotherapy
(E) progestin therapy

437. Fractional dilatation and curettage reveals endometrial carcinoma involving the cervix. This finding is

(A) of no prognostic significance
(B) of some prognostic significance but does not require change in management
(C) significant only if the cervical tumor is clinically obvious
(D) significant even if the disease is present only microscopically
(E) a contraindication for hysterectomy

438. The most common sarcoma of the uterus is

(A) endometrial stromal sarcoma
(B) carcinosarcoma
(C) leiomyosarcoma
(D) mixed mesodermal sarcoma
(E) rhabdomyosarcoma

439. Mixed mesodermal tumors of the uterus can be described by which of the following statements?

(A) They are more common than previously assumed and constitute about 17 to 18 percent of uterine malignancies
(B) Microscopic examination may reveal the presence of bone, cartilage, muscle, or other elements
(C) Their development has been associated with maternal intake of estrogen during pregnancy
(D) Five-year survival rate is quite good (approximately 80 percent)
(E) They are not known to occur before the menopausal years

440. The ovarian tumor most sensitive to radiation therapy is

(A) serous carcinoma
(B) mucinous carcinoma
(C) endometrioid carcinoma
(D) mesonephric carcinoma
(E) metastatic carcinoma

441. All of the following statements regarding ovarian cancer are true EXCEPT that

(A) it is the most common gynecological cancer
(B) it has the highest mortality rate among the common gynecological cancers
(C) it tends to be asymptomatic until it has reached an advanced stage
(D) its development may be influenced by environmental, cultural, or socioeconomic factors
(E) Papanicolaou (Pap) smears are ineffective for routine diagnostic screening

442. A 45-year-old woman has undergone a total abdominal hysterectomy and bilateral salpingo-oophorectomy for stage II serous carcinoma of the ovary. The most effective postoperative radiotherapeutic treatment of this woman would be

(A) pelvic irradiation
(B) vaginal radium insertion and pelvic irradiation
(C) whole-abdomen irradiation
(D) whole-abdomen and pelvic irradiation
(E) intraperitoneal radioisotope therapy

443. A 42-year-old multiparous woman comes to your office complaining of irregular menses and frequent urination. Her pregnancy test is negative. Ultrasonography and physical examination suggest the presence of a fibroid uterus (i.e., leiomyoma of the uterus) that is twice normal size. An examination performed 6 months earlier revealed a normal-size uterus. A hysterectomy would be recommended because

(A) a fibroid uterus leads to abnormal bleeding
(B) a fibroid the size of a 2-month pregnancy must be removed
(C) fibroids have a high malignant potential
(D) urinary frequency suggests severe pressure symptoms
(E) rapid appearance of fibroids warrants the procedure

444. A 25-year-old woman complains of diarrhea and weight loss; her heart rate is 130 per minute. Head, neck and chest x-rays, upper gastrointestinal series, small-bowel follow-through, and barium enema all are negative. An ovarian lesion, discovered during laparotomy, is biopsied (a photomicrograph of a specimen is shown below) and excised. After her tumor was removed, the woman's symptoms disappeared. The most likely diagnosis is

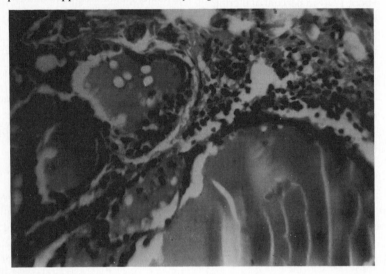

(A) carcinoid tumor
(B) dysgerminoma
(C) embryonal teratoma
(D) endometriosis
(E) struma ovarii

445. Women who have endometrial carcinoma most frequently present with which of the following symptoms?

(A) Bloating
(B) Weight loss
(C) Postmenopausal bleeding
(D) Vaginal discharge
(E) Hemoptysis

446. A patient in her first trimester of pregnancy is diagnosed with invasive cervical cancer. Treatment would include

(A) waiting until after delivery before treatment
(B) frequent pap smears through gestation
(C) termination of the pregnancy and concomitant or subsequent radiation or surgery as soon as possible
(D) delivery by cesarean section at term
(E) radiation only

447. Young women whose mothers took diethylstilbestrol (DES) during pregnancy are most likely to develop which of the following vaginal carcinomas?

(A) Papillary adenocarcinoma
(B) Squamous carcinoma
(C) Carcinoma of the infantile vagina
(D) Adenosquamous carcinoma
(E) Clear cell adenocarcinoma

448. The class of chemotherapeutic agents that is most effective in the management of women who have recurrent endometrial carcinoma is

(A) antimetabolites
(B) hormones
(C) alkylating agents
(D) Vinca alkaloids
(E) antibiotics

449. Melanoma of the vulva

(A) constitutes 2 to 9 percent of most series of vulvar cancer
(B) occurs mostly in the fifth decade
(C) occurs mostly in premenopausal women
(D) has an overall survival rate of 70 percent
(E) is nonaggressive

450. Women who have ovarian carcinoma most commonly present with which of the following symptoms?

(A) Vaginal bleeding and anorexia
(B) Weight loss and dyspareunia
(C) Nausea and vaginal discharge
(D) Constipation and frequent urination
(E) Abdominal distension and pain

451. The major mode of spread of ovarian neoplasms is by way of

(A) ovarian veins
(B) ovarian vein lymphatics
(C) pelvic lymphatics
(D) local extension
(E) peritoneal seeding

452. A 54-year-old woman undergoes a laparotomy because of a pelvic mass, which proves to be a unilateral ovarian neoplasm accompanied by a large omental metastasis. The most appropriate intraoperative course of action would be

(A) omental biopsy
(B) ovarian biopsy
(C) excision of the omental metastasis and unilateral oophorectomy
(D) omentectomy and bilateral salpingo-oophorectomy
(E) omentectomy, total abdominal hysterectomy, and bilateral salpingo-oophorectomy

453. Most deaths from cervical carcinoma can be attributed to

(A) local extension
(B) metastasis to the central nervous system
(C) metastasis to the liver and lungs
(D) iatrogenic causes
(E) none of the above

454. A woman is found to have a unilateral, invasive vulvar carcinoma that is 2 cm in diameter but that is not associated with evidence of lymph-node spread. Initial management of this woman most likely would consist of

(A) chemotherapy
(B) radiation therapy
(C) simple vulvectomy
(D) radical vulvectomy
(E) radical vulvectomy and bilateral inguinal lymphadenectomy

455. An exenteration procedure for recurrent cervical cancer would include all of the following EXCEPT

(A) removal of the bladder
(B) removal of the uterus
(C) removal of the symphysis
(D) removal of the rectum
(E) removal of the pelvic nodes

---

456. A 55-year-old woman has a 3-cm raised irregular white lesion at the mucocutaneous junction of the vulva. A sample of the biopsied lesion is shown below. The most likely diagnosis is

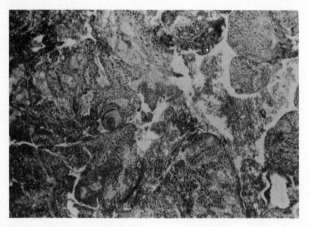

(A) tuberculosis
(B) Bowen's disease
(C) Paget's disease
(D) invasive squamous cell carcinoma
(E) fibrosarcoma

457. The neoplasm most sensitive to appropriate chemotherapy is

(A) gestational trophoblastic disease
(B) ovarian dysgerminoma
(C) Burkitt's lymphoma
(D) endometrial carcinoma
(E) ovarian serous carcinoma

458. The ovarian cyst or tumor that is most common during infancy and childhood is

(A) dermoid cyst
(B) theca-lutein cyst
(C) giant follicle cyst
(D) granuloma cell tumor
(E) benign solid teratoma

459. All of the following statements about Brenner tumors of the ovary are true EXCEPT that

(A) they generally are benign
(B) they are characterized microscopically by areas of epithelial cells surrounded by mesenchymal tissue
(C) their cells have a characteristic "coffee-bean" nucleus
(D) they tend to grow rather slowly
(E) they rarely are larger than 2 cm in diameter

460. A 43-year-old multiparous woman has a 4-year history of irregular menses and frequent urination. Physical examination reveals an irregular uterus that is two or three times normal size. As the woman's physician, you now would

(A) perform a dilatation and curettage
(B) order a pregnancy test
(C) order ultrasonography
(D) order intravenous pyelography
(E) schedule a hysterectomy

461. A 48-year-old woman presents with a nontender fluctuant mass in her right vulva that causes some discomfort when walking and during coitus and that is consistent with a diagnosis of Bartholin's cyst. What is the most appropriate treatment?

(A) Marsupialization
(B) Antibiotics
(C) Surgical excision
(D) Incision and drainage
(E) No treatment necessary

462. Carcinoma in situ of the cervix is characterized by all of the following EXCEPT

(A) involvement of the entire thickness of the squamous epithelium
(B) cells resembling those of invasive carcinoma
(C) evidence of stromal invasion
(D) complete loss of stratification
(E) occasional regression and disappearance

463. Paget's disease is characterized by all of the following statements EXCEPT that

(A) it occurs in the nipple and vulva
(B) local recurrences are common
(C) it is often associated with subajacent adenocarcinoma or squamous cell carcinoma
(D) it often stains darker than the surrounding keratinocytes
(E) surgery is the best treatment

464. Ovarian neoplasms most commonly arise from

(A) coelomic epithelium
(B) nonspecific mesenchyme
(C) specialized gonadal stroma
(D) primitive germ cells
(E) none of the above

465. An intravenous pyelogram showing hydronephrosis in the work-up of a cervical cancer otherwise confined to a normal size cervix would mean

(A) stage I
(B) stage II
(C) stage III
(D) stage IV
(E) none of the above

DIRECTIONS: Each question below contains four suggested answers of which **one or more** is correct. Choose the answer:

A	if	**1, 2, and 3**	are correct
B	if	**1 and 3**	are correct
C	if	**2 and 4**	are correct
D	if	**4**	is correct
E	if	**1, 2, 3, and 4**	are correct

466. Clinical symptoms that may be associated with hydatid mole include

(1) nausea and vomiting
(2) hypertension
(3) lower abdominal pain
(4) bleeding

467. True statements about clear cell adenocarcinoma of the cervix and vagina include which of the following?

(1) It has been related to prenatal DES exposure
(2) It shows a hobnail pattern on microscopic examination
(3) It usually appears as an exophytic lesion
(4) Affected women are best treated with radiotherapy

468. Adenocarcinoma of the endometrium can be described by which of the following statements?

(1) It is primarily a disease of postmenopausal women
(2) The average age of affected women is 10 years more than the average age of women who have cervical carcinoma
(3) It has a more favorable prognosis than cervical cancer, with the 5-year survival rate approaching 75 percent
(4) It is increasing in frequency relative to carcinoma of the cervix

469. The spread of adenocarcinoma of the body of the uterus can be described by which of the following statements?

(1) Distant organs, such as the liver, are frequently involved
(2) Dissemination is chiefly by way of the lymphatics
(3) The tumor resembles cervical carcinoma in its frequency of dissemination
(4) Direct extension is an important route of dissemination

470. A patient presents with a Pap smear showing mild dysplasia. The next steps in management would include

(1) hysterectomy
(2) repeat Pap smear
(3) cone biopsy
(4) colposcopy

471. Important prognostic factors concerning ovarian epithelial carcinoma include

(1) extent of the tumor
(2) volume of the tumor
(3) histological differentiation of the tumor
(4) presence of ascites

SUMMARY OF DIRECTIONS

A	B	C	D	E
1,2,3 only	1,3 only	2,4 only	4 only	All are correct

472. Cervical carcinoma is considered invasive when there is

(1) a breakthrough of the basement membrane
(2) penetration of the stroma
(3) involvement of the lymphatics
(4) involvement of the endocervical glands

473. Which of the following statements can characterize epidermoid carcinoma of the vulva?

(1) It is associated with an increased incidence of epidermoid carcinoma of the endocervix
(2) It is seen less frequently than adenocarcinoma
(3) It tends to develop in women who are older than those affected by adenocarcinoma
(4) It tends to be more advanced when diagnosed than adenocarcinoma

474. Carcinoma of the fallopian tube can be described by which of the following statements?

(1) It is an uncommon lesion, accounting for approximately 0.2 to 0.5 percent of primary genital-tract malignancies
(2) Bilateral involvement occurs in approximately 50 percent of affected patients
(3) Its microscopic appearance can be papillary or papillary-alveolar
(4) It is considered only mildly malignant and is associated with a good 5-year survival rate

475. Non-neoplastic cysts of the ovary include

(1) theca-lutein cysts
(2) pregnancy luteoma
(3) endometriotic cysts
(4) corpus luteum cysts

476. Dermoid cysts of the ovary can be characterized by which of the following statements?

(1) They often contain bone and teeth, which may be seen on abdominal x-ray
(2) They may be associated with severe chemical peritonitis if ruptured
(3) They are often pedunculated
(4) They are on rare occasions associated with hemolytic anemia

477. Women who have which of the following characteristics are at high risk for endometrial carcinoma?

(1) Hypertension
(2) Diabetes
(3) Obesity
(4) Familial history of endometrial carcinoma

478. Evidence in evaluating cell types found in carcinoma of the endometrium suggests that

(1) poorly differentiated adenocarcinomas have a poor prognosis
(2) adenoacanthomas have a poor prognosis
(3) adenosquamous carcinomas have a poor prognosis
(4) adenosquamous tumors occur more often in young women

479. For the management of women who have endometrial carcinoma, intracavitary radium has been employed routinely

(1) as a treatment for women who have ovarian metastases
(2) as a treatment for women who have vaginal apical recurrences
(3) as a treatment for women who have metastases of the pelvic sidewall
(4) as primary therapy for inoperable patients

480. True statements about mucinous carcinoma of the ovary include which of the following?

(1) It usually is diagnosed at a less advanced stage than serous carcinoma
(2) It tends to be unilateral
(3) It tends to be well differentiated
(4) Affected women have a 50-percent chance of surviving 5 years

481. Lichen sclerosis is characterized by

(1) blunting or loss of the rete ridges
(2) development of a homogeneous subepithelial layer in the dermis
(3) a band of chronic inflammatory infiltrate below the dermis
(4) an increase in the number of cellular layers in the epidermis

482. Sarcoma botryoides can be characterized by which of the following statements?

(1) It tends to be multicentric
(2) Its initial manifestation usually is lower abdominal pain
(3) It occurs most frequently in young girls
(4) Cartilaginous and osseous elements are common

483. Meigs syndrome can be described by which of the following statements?

(1) Hydrothorax and ascites are the primary features
(2) It rarely is seen in combination with ovarian fibromas
(3) It can occur with Brenner tumor, thecoma, and granulosa cell tumor
(4) It characteristically is associated with large subserous myomas

SUMMARY OF DIRECTIONS

A	B	C	D	E
1,2,3 only	1,3 only	2,4 only	4 only	All are correct

484. True statements regarding myomas of the uterus include which of the following?

(1) They are the most common benign tumors of the uterus
(2) Sarcomatous change is frequent in women over 50 years of age who have myomas
(3) Carneous or red degeneration of myomas occurs frequently during pregnancy
(4) Myomas tend to grow more rapidly after the menopause

485. True statements about ovarian neoplasms in children include which of the following?

(1) They are most often of germ cell origin
(2) They are an infrequent cause of precocious puberty
(3) Coelomic epithelial tumors are usually benign
(4) Tumors of germ cell origin are frequently malignant

486. Epithelial ovarian tumors of low potential malignancy (borderline malignancies) can be described by which of the following statements?

(1) They represent nearly half of all epithelial ovarian tumors
(2) They occasionally are associated with late recurrences and death
(3) They seldom, if ever, metastasize within the peritoneal cavity
(4) They are not associated with destructive infiltration of the ovarian stroma

487. Serous carcinoma of the ovary can be characterized by which of the following statements?

(1) It is the most common epithelial carcinoma of the ovary
(2) It often contains psammoma bodies
(3) It is bilateral in approximately one-third of affected women
(4) It frequently is associated with pelvic endometriosis

488. Characteristics of paraovarian cysts include which of the following?

(1) They rise from mesonephric duct remnants
(2) They rarely reach considerable size
(3) They can often be removed without damage to the ovary and tube
(4) They grow outside the leaves of the broad ligament

489. Vaginal carcinoma in women whose mothers received DES during pregnancy can be characterized by which of the following statements?

(1) It is most commonly located in the middle and outer portions of the vagina
(2) It classically occurs in women in their teens and early twenties
(3) Electron microscopy has shown that it is müllerian in origin
(4) It occurs in less than 0.1 percent of women exposed in utero to DES

490. Epithelial neoplasms of the ovary can be of which of the following histological types?

(1) Serous
(2) Mucinous
(3) Endometrioid
(4) Mesonephroid

491. Studies show that cervical cancer is associated with

(1) early first coitus
(2) incidence of cigarette smoking
(3) multiparity
(4) use of oral contraceptives

DIRECTIONS: The groups of questions below consist of lettered choices followed by several numbered items. For each numbered item select the **one** lettered choice with which it is **most** closely associated. Each lettered choice may be used once, more than once, or not at all.

Questions 492–496

For each description that follows, select the ovarian tumor with which it is most likely to be associated.

(A) Granulosa tumor
(B) Sertoli-Leydig cell tumor
(C) Immature teratoma
(D) Gonadoblastoma
(E) Krukenberg's tumor

492. Frequently associated with virilization

493. Frequently associated with endometrial carcinoma

494. Tends to recur more than 5 years following the original diagnosis

495. Calcifications present on pelvic radiographs

496. Correlation between malignant potential and the amount of embryogenic tissue

Questions 497–500

Match the ovarian tumors listed below with the micrograph that correctly exemplifies it.

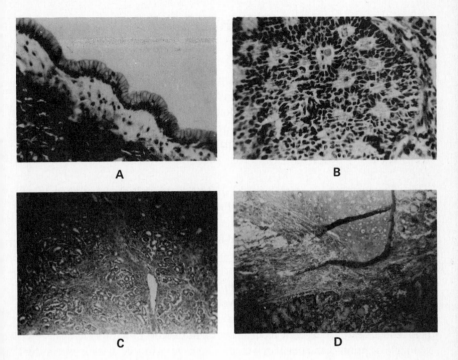

(A) Slide **A**
(B) Slide **B**
(C) Slide **C**
(D) Slide **D**
(E) None of the above

97. Granulosa cell tumor

98. Arrhenoblastoma

99. Benign cystic teratoma

00. Mucinous cystadenoma

Benign and Malignant Neoplasms

Answers

434. The answer is D. *(Morrow, ed 2. pp 210–214.)* Endometrioid ovarian carcinoma accounts for about 15 percent of all ovarian carcinomas. It is indistinguishable from adenocarcinoma of endometrial origin. Squamous differentiation is common. Approximately 10 percent of endometrioid ovarian cancer is accompanied by ovarian endometriosis, but malignant transformation has not been demonstrated.

435. The answer is B. *(Morrow, ed 2. p 7.)* According to the International Federation of Gynecology and Obstetrics (FIGO) classification, stage I is carcinoma confined to the corpus, stage II is involvement of the corpus and cervix, stage III is extension beyond the uterus but limited to the true pelvis, and stage IV involves extension outside the true pelvis.

436. The answer is C. *(DiSaia, ed 2. pp 161–167.)* Hysterectomy is the primary mode of treatment for women who have endometrial carcinoma confined to the uterine corpus. External beam and intracavitary radiation have been employed to help reduce central and pelvic recurrences of the cancer. Progestin therapy is used routinely as primary treatment of women who have advanced disease or recurrent carcinoma, and chemotherapy is used for patients whose tumors have failed to respond to other forms of therapy.

437. The answer is D. *(DiSaia, ed 2. pp 149–151.)* Endometrial carcinoma involving the cervix is significant even if present only as microscopic disease. The lymphatic drainage of the uterine corpus is primarily by way of the lymphatics that follow the ovarian vessels. Because involvement of the cervix allows the cancer to metatasize via the parametrial lymphatics, 5-year survival rate is reduced (regardless of the volume of tumor present) and intense radiotherapeutic treatment is required. Hysterectomy need not be excluded from the management program.

438. The answer is D. *(DiSaia, ed 2. pp 182–184.)* Mixed mesodermal sarcomas are most common. They are discovered most frequently during a histological examination of a leiomyomatous uterus and are often clinically and grossly indistinguishable from benign leiomyoma. A rapid enlargement of a leiomyomatous uterus and may be the only indication of the presence of a sarcoma.

439. The answer is B. *(Novak, ed 8. pp 300–305.)* Mixed mesodermal tumors (mesenchymomas) of the uterus are similar to endometrial sarcoma. They are made up of a composite of mesodermal elements such as bone, cartilage, and muscle. The combined incidence of these two types of malignancy is no higher than 0.5 percent of all gynecological malignancies. Although mixed mesodermal tumors occur most frequently in postmenopausal women, one variant, sarcoma botryoides, can develop in young children. Prognosis is poor, with a 5-year survival rate of 26 to 28 percent being the highest reported. Maternal ingestion of estrogen during pregnancy has not, as yet, been associated with the development of mixed mesodermal tumors.

440. The answer is C. *(Green, ed 3. p 497.)* In general, epithelial ovarian tumors are radiosensitive, but the endometrioid tumor is most sensitive.

441. The answer is A. *(DeSaia, ed 2. pp 288–298.)* Ovarian carcinoma, though the third most common malignancy of gynecological origin (after endometrial and cervical carcinoma), is associated with the highest mortality rate among the common gynecological malignancies. The inability of routine screening tests to diagnose this malignancy in an early stage, in contrast to the efficacy of the Papanicolaou (Pap) smear in detecting cervical cancer, is chiefly responsible for the high mortality rate. Most patients have advanced disease by the time their symptoms appear. Environmental, cultural, socioeconomic, and dietary factors all may play a role in the development of ovarian cancer.

442. The answer is D. *(Novak, ed 8. p 549.)* Postoperative whole-abdomen irradiation combined with additional radiation to the pelvis has produced the highest 5-year survival rates of any treatment used for patients who have stage II epithelial ovarian tumors. Because ovarian tumor cells tend to exfoliate and spread throughout the abdominal cavity, irradiation of the pelvis alone is insufficient treatment. The liver and kidneys must be shielded during at least part of the external beam therapy, and bowel injury may be a late sequela.

443. The answer is E. *(Kistner, ed 3. pp 231–232. Romney, ed 2. p 1085.)* A rapid growth in fibroids (leiomyomas), persistent bleeding, or a fibroid of 12-weeks gestational size or more is considered a valid indication for hysterectomy. Fibroids have a low malignant potential, rarely cause significant pressure when small, and may not cause bleeding problems even when left untreated. They are the most common benign tumors in women and are five times more frequent in blacks than whites.

444. The answer is E. *(Novak, ed 8. pp 490–494.)* The tissue specimen that accompanies the question represents struma ovarii, which is composed of aberrant thyroid tissue that is frequently active and which is associated with mature cystic teratomas. The woman described manifests symptoms of thyrotoxicosis, such as diarrhea, rapid pulse, and weight loss; though not reported, her serum thyroxine levels would be elevated. The pathological picture is characterized by thyroid tissue with large acini filled with colloid.

445. The answer is C. *(Jones, ed 10. p 411.)* Postmenopausal bleeding is the most common presenting symptom of women who have endometrial carcinoma. Because this warning signal is present even in the earliest stage of the disease, early diagnosis and treatment are possible. In fact, approximately 70 percent of affected women have stage I disease when they first seek treatment.

446. The answer is C. *(Green, ed 3. p 439.)* Patients in their first trimester should receive treatment immediately. Radiation or radical surgery can be done at the time of termination or immediately following. In the third trimester the infant can be delivered via cesarean section and treatment begun as soon as possible. Vaginal deliveries are contraindicated for fear of disseminating the tumor.

447. The answer is E. *(DiSaia, ed 2. pp 237–251.)* Young women whose mothers ingested diethylstilbestrol (DES) during pregnancy are more apt to develop clear cell adenocarcinoma than other types of vaginal carcinoma. Although squamous carcinomas are the most common tumors of the vagina, they usually occur in women over 40 years of age. Two rare vaginal carcinomas are papillary adenocarcinoma, which primarily affects older women, and carcinoma of the infantile vagina, which histologically resembles an endodermal sinus tumor of the ovary. Adenosquamous carcinomas usually are found in the uterus and less frequently in the cervix.

448. The answer is B. *(DiSaia, ed 2. pp 172–173.)* Progestins have been employed successfully in the treatment of women who have recurrent endometrial carcinoma. In many series, response rates of 30 to 40 percent have been noted. The most frequently employed agents have been hydroxyprogesterone caproate (Delalutin) and medroxyprogesterone acetate (Provera). Single-agent chemotherapy with nonhormonal agents has produced disappointing responses in patients affected by advanced or recurrent endometrial carcinoma.

449. The answer is A. *(Blaustein, ed 2. pp 48–49.)* Melanoma of the vulva constitutes 2 to 9 percent of vulvar cancer. The mean age of incidence is 54, and most cases occur in the sixth and seventh decades, although 32 percent are premenopausal. It is highly aggressive, and the overall survival rate is only 30 percent.

450. The answer is E. *(Morrow, ed 2. p 192.)* Approximately 50 percent of women who have ovarian cancer present with abdominal distension, and 50 percent present with abdominal pain. Gastrointestinal symptoms, which occur in about 20 percent of affected women, often are secondary to the development of ascites. Urinary-tract symptoms, due to the pressure exerted by a rapidly growing mass, and abnormal vaginal bleeding are the initial symptoms of ovarian cancer in 15 percent of affected women.

451. The answer is E. *(DiSaia, ed 2. p 301.)* Peritoneal seeding is the major mode of spread of ovarian neoplasms. Ovarian malignancies also may extend locally to adjoining structures, such as the uterus, fallopian tubes, pelvic peritoneum, bladder peritoneum, and serosa of the sigmoid colon. Although dissemination by lymphatic and hematogenous routes does occur, it is of lesser importance than peritoneal seeding in producing symptoms and eventually causing death.

452. The answer is E. *(Morrow, ed 2. pp 197–200.)* The survivability of women who have ovarian carcinoma varies inversely with the amount of residual tumor left after the initial surgery. At the time of laparotomy, a maximum effort should be made to determine the sites of tumor spread and excise all resectable tumor. Although the uterus and ovary may appear grossly normal, there is a relatively high incidence of occult metastases to these organs; for this reason, they should be removed during the initial surgery.

453. The answer is A. *(Novak, ed 8. p 130.)* Most deaths from cervical cancer result from the effects of local extension. These effects include urinary insufficiency, intestinal obstruction, and debility and malnutrition. Approximately two-fifths of all women who die of cervical cancer have evidence of extrapelvic metastasis; spread of the tumor, presumably via the bloodstream, occasionally involves distant organs, including the liver, spine, and brain.

454. The answer is E. *(Morrow, ed 2. pp 298–300.)* Women who have invasive vulvar carcinoma usually are treated surgically. If the lesions are unilateral, are not associated with fixed or ulcerated inguinal lymph nodes, and do not involve the urethra, vagina, anus, or rectum, then treatment usually consists of radical vulvectomy and bilateral inguinal lymphadenectomy. If inguinal lymph nodes show evidence of metastatic disease, bilateral pelvic lymphadenectomy is usually performed. Radiation therapy, though not a routine part of the management of women who have early vulvar carcinoma, is employed (as an alternative to pelvic exenteration with radical vulvectomy) in the treatment of women who have local advanced carcinoma.

455. The answer is C. *(Novak, ed 10. p 345.)* Exenteration is a radical procedure for recurrent cervical cancer in only those cases where the lymph nodes are negative. It involves removal of all pelvic structures except the bone and musculature.

456. The answer is D. *(Novak, ed 8. pp 43–48.)* The woman described in the question has invasive squamous cell carcinoma of the vulva, with penetration below the basement membrane. The squamous epithelial cells have an irregular shape and an abnormal nuclear-cytoplasmic ratio and show an increased number of mitotic figures. Tuberculosis of the vulva is characterized by multinucleated giant cells; Bowen's disease tissue does not show invasion below the basement membrane; and Paget's disease of the vulva, which is rare, is characterized by Paget cells, large cells that have abundant granular cytoplasm and basophilic nuclei.

457. The answer is A. *(DiSaia, ed 2. pp 200–211.)* Gestational trophoblastic disease is the neoplasm most sensitive to appropriate chemotherapeutic agents, such as methotrexate and acitinomycin D. Treatment of women who have nonmetastatic gestational trophoblastic disease is almost 100 percent successful and allows reproductive function to be preserved. Cure rates for metastatic disease approach 90 percent.

458. The answer is A. *(Green, ed 3. pp 126-127.)* Different types of ovarian cancer predominate at different stages of a woman's life. For example, adenocarcinomas, which occur primarily in postmenopausal women, are very rare in infants and children. Benign solid teratomas and especially dermoid cysts, on the other hand, make up about half of the ovarian neoplasms affecting young girls. Giant follicle cysts and teca-lutein cysts also occur rather frequently and presumably are due to maternal gonadotropin stimulation. Granulosa cell tumors, which develop before puberty in about 5 percent of cases, can be a cause of precocious puberty.

459. The answer is E. *(Novak, ed 8. pp 441-449.)* Brenner tumors of the ovary, which generally are benign, slow-growing, and asymptomatic, account for 1 to 2 percent of all ovarian neoplasms. Size varies widely; although many are microscopic, some may grow to be quite large [one tumor weighing more than 8.5 kg (19 lb) has been reported]. "Walthard rests," which are nests of epithelial cells surrounded by mesenchymal tissue, are diagnostic of Brenner tumor. Nuclei of the epithelial cells are grooved longitudinally and, as a result, are referred to as "coffee-bean" nuclei.

460. The answer is B. *(Kistner, ed 3. p 230.)* If a woman in the childbearing years has an enlarged uterus, a pregnancy test should be performed. Ultrasonography is a more expensive alternative; and an ultrasonogram may be difficult to interpret if both fibroids and an intrauterine pregnancy are present.

461. The answer is C. *(Blaustein, ed 2. p 26.)* Although rare, adenocarcinoma of Bartholin's gland has to be ruled out in women over 40 years of age who present with Bartholin's cyst. The appropriate treatment in these cases is surgical excision of the Bartholin's gland for a close pathological examination. In cases of abscess formation, both marsupialization of the sac and incision with drainage with appropriate antibiotics are accepted modes of therapy. In the case of the asymptomatic Bartholin's cyst, no treatment is necessary.

462. The answer is C. *(Novak, ed 8. pp 120–123.)* Carcinoma in situ (preinvasive cancer) of the cervix involves the entire squamous epithelium, which is displaced by cells that are similar to those of invasive carcinoma. Stratification is completely lost, but no evidence of stromal or lymphatic invasion has been noted. Although carcinoma in situ is generally considered to precede development of frank invasive cancer, the lesion has been reported to regress and disappear on occasion.

463. The answer is D. *(Blaustein, ed 2. pp 42–45.)* Paget cells often present singly or in nests, and their pale cytoplasm easily differentiates them from surrounding keratinocytes. Paget cells should be a clue to underlying breast carcinoma or squamous cell carcinoma of the genital region. It commonly occurs in the nipple and vulva and local recurrences are common. The recommended treatment is surgery.

464. The answer is A. *(Morrow, ed 2. pp 201–202.)* Ovarian neoplasms arise more commonly from coelomic epithelium than from any other source. Many tumors of this group include epithelium that histologically resembles endocervical, endometrial, or fallopian-tube epithelium (giving rise respectively to mucinous, endometroid, and serous carcinomas). Other, less common ovarian tumors of coelomic epithelial origin include mesonephroid carcinoma, Brenner tumors, mixed mesodermal tumors, and carcinosarcomas. Epithelial tumors frequently contain mixed cell types; categorization of these tumors is according to the cell type that predominates.

465. The answer is C. *(Morrow, ed 2. p 78.)* A positive IVP would mean extension to the pelvic side wall and thus a stage III carcinoma, specifically stage IIIb.

466. The answer is E (all). *(Morrow, ed 2. p 329.)* Hydatid moles are suspected and diagnosed by symptoms that include nausea and vomiting, hypertension from toxemia, lower abdominal pain, and bleeding. Further data include uterine size large for dates and a characteristic honeycomb pattern on ultrasound. Karyotype of molar tissue reveals 46,XX.

467. The answer is A (1, 2, 3). *(Green, ed 3. pp 128–131.)* In the late 1960s, a surprisingly large number of cases of a rare type of clear cell adenocarcinoma of the cervix and vagina were discovered in Boston. Careful epidemiological investigation revealed that nearly all the mothers of affected girls had taken DES or a similar drug during pregnancy. These tumors are exophytic lesions that are friable and red. Microscopic examination characteristically reveals the presence of cystic spaces lined with so-called hobnail cells. Because affected women usually are in their adolescence and because the tumors are relatively radioresistant, surgery has been the main component of management.

468. The answer is E (all). *(Novak, ed 8. pp 204–205.)* Although the carcinogenes of endometrial cancer is still in dispute, several facts regarding its incidence are clear. The disease primarily affects women who have passed the menopause; on the average, endometrial cancer appears 10 years later than the onset of cervical carcinoma. The fact that the frequency of this condition has been increasing certainly is due in part to the increased life span of American women. Most studies have revealed a 5-year survival rate of about 75 percent for women who have endometrial cancer.

469. The answer is C (2, 4). *(Novak, ed 8, p 219.)* Although the most common route of dissemination of adenocarcinoma of the body of the uterus is the lymphatics, this tumor spreads much less often than cervical malignancies and only rarely affects distant organs. Nearby surface structures are affected more frequently, and the cervix, bladder, and rectum can become involved in advanced cases. Direct extension, though not as common as lymphatic dissemination, also is important.

470. The answer is C (2, 4). *(Blaustein, ed 2. pp 172–173.)* Management would require a repeat Pap smear and biopsies to rule out invasive disease before any treatment is undertaken, especially the more invasive procedures. The biopsies should be colposcopically directed.

471. The answer is E (all). *(Morrow, ed 2. pp 231–232.)* The extent (or stage) and the volume of a tumor are probably the most important prognostic considerations in the management of women who have ovarian epithelial carcinoma. However, on a stage-for-stage basis, women who have well-differentiated tumors have better prognoses than women who have poorly differentiated tumors. The presence of ascites or peritoneal washings that are cytologically positive for malignant cells decreases the 5-year survival of affected women.

472. The answer is A (1, 2, 3). *(Novak, ed 8. pp 123–129.)* Carcinoma of the cervix is considered to be invasive when the basement membrane has been pierced, allowing cancer cells into the stroma. Histological evidence of abnormal cell maturation and presence of cancer cells in the lymphatics also indicates invasive disease. Involvement of endocervical glands is not indicative of invasion.

473. The answer is B (1, 3). *(Morrow, ed 2. pp 287–288.)* Epidermoid carcinoma, the most common variety of vulvar cancer, usually is diagnosed at a less advanced stage than adenocarcinoma, which is a rare tumor that most often arises from Bartholin's glands. Epidermoid carcinoma tends to affect women who, on the average, are older than those affected by adenocarcinoma. Women who have epidermoid carcinoma of the vulva have been noted to have an increased incidence of epidermoid carcinoma of the cervix.

474. The answer is B (1, 3). *(Novak, ed 8. pp 335–341.)* Because affected women have a low 5-year survival rate, primary tubal carcinoma is thought to be highly malignant; this relationship, however, may be due more to delayed discovery of the tumor than to its malignant potential. Primary tubal carcinoma accounts for only 0.2 to 0.5 percent of primary malignancies of the genital tract. Microscopically, these tumors present a papillary or papillary-alveolar pattern. Bilateral involvement occurs in about one-fourth of affected women.

475. The answer is E (all). *(Morrow, ed 2. p 188.)* Corpus luteum cysts represent normal functional cysts. Theca-lutein cysts are follicular cysts with luteinization of the thecal cells. Pregnancy luteoma is a nodular hyperplasia of ovarian lutein cells. Endometriotic cysts are the result of cyclic hemorrhage into a focus of ovarian endometriosis.

476. The answer is E (all). *(Green, ed 3. pp 476–477.)* Dermoid cysts are characteristically pedunculated, which predisposes them to undergo tension, one of the more common complications associated with this tumor. It has been estimated that teeth, which are visible on abdominal x-ray, are present in approximately 50 percent of cases. When the dermoid cyst is ruptured, the contents are extremely irritating to the peritoneum and incite an intense granulomatous inflammatory reaction. Hemolytic anemia has been reported as one of the complications; it resolves completely on surgical removal of the dermoid cyst.

477. The answer is E (all). *(DiSaia, ed 2. pp 146–147.)* Endometrial carcinoma tends to occur in obese, diabetic women who undergo late-onset menopause and are nulliparous or have low parity. Other factors that may predispose to endometrial carcinoma include hypertension, cancer at other sites (e.g., ovary and breast), and familial history of this malignancy.

478. The answer is B (1, 3). *(Jones, ed 10. pp 405–410.)* Recent evidence suggests that adenosquamous carcinoma of the endometrium has a poorer prognosis than either adenocarcinoma or adenoacanthoma of the endometrium. It has yet to be resolved whether the poorer prognosis associated with adenosquamous lesions is due to the population of malignant squamous cells or to the poorly differentiated adenomatous elements, which normally carry a poor prognosis. Adenoacanthoma, which is characterized by benign metaplasia of squamous epithelium, has a prognosis similar to that of other adenocarcinomas of the endometrium. Adenosquamous tumors tend to occur more frequently in older women.

479. The answer is C (2, 4). *(DiSaia, ed 2. p 167.)* Intracavitary radium has been successfully employed as the primary mode of therapy for women who have surgically inoperable endometrial cancer and have small uteri with a well-differentiated tumor. Vaginal apical recurrences occur in 10 to 15 percent of affected women who were treated by hysterectomy alone; this incidence can be reduced significantly with the use of intravaginal radium. Because the effectiveness of intracavitary radium rapidly decreases as tissue depth increases, it is not a satisfactory treatment for women who have ovarian or pelvic sidewall metastases.

480. The answer is E (all). *(Blaustein, ed 2. pp 529–530.)* Mucinous carcinomas of the ovary usually are diagnosed at an earlier stage than serous carcinomas and tend to be histologically well differentiated. This combination of diagnosis at an early stage (when the tumors frequently are unilateral) and well-differentiated histological appearance is probably the reason that women who have mucinous carcinoma have a better 5-year survival rate than women affected by serous carcinoma. Mucinous tumors of the ovary, which are less common than serous lesions, usually are lobulated and may grow to enormous proportions.

481. The answer is A (1, 2, 3). *(Blaustein, ed 2. pp 37–39.)* This condition was formerly termed lichen sclerosis et atrophicus, but recent studies have precluded that atrophy exists. Mitotic figures are rare, however. There is an associated decrease in the number of cellular layers as well as a loss in the number of melanocytes. Mechanical trauma has produced bullous areas of lymphedema and lacunae filled with erythrocytes, and ulcerations may be seen. It is not a premalignant lesion.

482. The answer is B (1, 3). *(Morrow, ed 2. pp 282–283. Romney, ed 2. p 379.)* Sarcoma botryoides, a rare and highly malignant tumor, is characterized grossly by a polypoid mass than can expand to occupy the entire vagina and frequently protrudes through the vaginal introitus. The usual presenting symptom is vaginal discharge or bleeding. Sarcoma botryoides, which occurs most frequently in young girls, is usually multicentric in origin. Cartilagenous and osseous elements are not commonly found, although rhabdomyoblastic elements are. Extensive surgery (extenteration), without which death will result, can extend the survival rate to several years.

483. The answer is B (1, 3). *(Novak, ed 8. pp 451–454.)* Hydrothorax and ascites are the characteristic features of Meigs syndrome. It is believed that fluid accumulates in the thorax by permeating through diaphragmatic lymphatics. First described in association with ovarian fibromas, Meigs syndrome also can be seen in combination with Brenner tumors, thecomas, granulosa cell tumors, and other solid ovarian tumors; large subserous myomas, however, are not associated with development of this syndrome.

484. The answer is B (1, 3). *(Green, ed 3. pp 381–385–387.)* Myomas are indeed the most common benign gynecological tumor in women. It has been estimated that approximately 20 to 30 percent of all women will develop this tumor during their lifetime, with many of them remaining completely asymptomatic. The incidence has been shown to be higher in black women for yet-unknown reasons. Sarcomatous changes are infrequent, being in the range of approximately 0.5 percent. Red or carneous degeneration of myomas occurs especially during pregnancy. When the high levels of estrogen stimulate rapid growth of the tumor, resulting in impairment of the vascular supply, especially to the center of the tumor. Clinically, it is important to distinguish between this entity and other possible causes of abdominal pain in pregnancy since conservative supportive therapy usually suffices in the case of red degeneration of myomas. Following the menopause, the myomas usually decrease in size because of decreased estrogen levels.

485. The answer is E (all). *(Morrow, ed 2. p 257–259.)* Most ovarian neoplasms in children are of germ cell origin, and about half of these tumors are malignant. Functioning ovarian tumors have been reported to produce precocious puberty in about 2 percent of affected patients. Epithelial tumors of the ovary, which are quite rare in prepubertal girls, are benign in approximately 90 percent of all cases.

486. The answer is C (2, 4). *(Morrow, ed 2. pp 207–208.)* Epithelial ovarian tumors of low potential malignancy represent 15 percent of all epithelial ovarian tumors. Although they do not infiltrate destructively into the ovarian stroma, these borderline malignancies have been associated with late recurrences and death and may metastasize throughout the peritoneal cavity. Histologically, these tumors demonstrate proliferateive activity, abnormal mitoses, and nuclear abnormalities. Ten-year survival rates of women who have stage I tumors of low potential malignancy have been reported to be 95 percent.

487. The answer is A (1, 2, 3). *(Morrow, ed 2. pp 208–209.)* Serous carcinoma is the most common epithelial tumor of the ovary. Psammoma bodies can be seen in approximately 30 percent of these tumors; and bilateral involvement charcterizes about one-third of all serous carcinomas. Although mesonephroid carcinomas tend to be associated with pelvic endometriosis, a similar association has not been demonstrated for serous carcinomas.

488. The answer is B (1, 3). *(Green, ed 3. p 475.)* These mesonephric duct remnant cysts should always be considered in the differential diagnosis of any cystic adnexal mass. They often reach sizes large enough to fill the entire pelvis. Although they displace and distort the ovary and tube, they can be removed without significant damage to either. The ureter must be protected when dissecting in the broad ligament.

489. The answer is E (all). *(Novak, ed 8, pp 73–74.)* A number of young women whose mothers were treated with DES during pregnancy (particularly before the eighteenth week of gestation) have been found to have andenocarcinoma of the vagina. The tumors of these women, who generally are in their late teens or early twenties, usually are located in the middle third or outer third of the vagina. Microscopic examination reveals that the malignancies are clear cell tumors with papillary projections; when viewed by electon microscopy, these tumors show evidence of a müllerian origin.

490. The answer is E (all). *(Novak, ed 8. pp 396–435.)* Epithelial neoplasms, which comprise 75 to 80 percent of all primary ovarian cancers, may be of the following histological types: seros, mucinous, endometroid, and mesonephroid. These types may be thought of as forms of differentiated mesotheliomas. Serous lesions are the most common variety of ovarian cystomas. Mucinous tumors may become large enough to fill the abdomen. The prognosis is good for women who have endometrioid lesions, which metastasize only infrequently, and are not considered to be very malignant. Pure mesonephroid tumors are rare.

491. The answer is B (1, 3). *(Novak, ed 10. pp 297–301.)* The main risk factors of cervical cancer include early exposure to coitus, especially with multiple partners, multiparity, and infection with herpes simplex virus type 2 and other viruses. The role of oral contraceptives has not been established.

492–496. The answers are: 492-B, 493-A, 494-A, 495-D, 496-C. *(Morrow, ed 2. pp 244, 249–252. Romney, ed 2. p 1167. Rutledge, pp 206–207.)* Sertoli-Leydig cell tumors, which represent less than 1 percent of ovarian tumors, may produce symptoms of virilization. Histologically, they resemble fetal testes; clinically, they must be distinguished from other functioning ovarian neoplasms as well as from tumors of the adrenal glands. Recurrences of Sertoli-Leydig cell tumors, which seem to have a low malignant potential, usually appear within 3 years of the original diagnosis.

Granulosa and theca cell tumors often are associated with excessive estrogen production, which may cause pseudoprecocious puberty, postmenopausal bleeding, or menorrhagia. These tumors are associated with endometrial carcinoma in 15 percent of patients. Because these tumors are quite friable, affected women frequently present with symptoms caused by tumor rupture and intraperitoneal bleeding. Granulosa tumors are low-grade malignancies that tend to recur more than 5 years after the initial diagnosis. Because their malignant potential is impossible to predict histologically, long-term follow-up is mandatory for these patients. Recurrences have been reported as late as 33 years after the original diagnosis.

Gonadoblastomas frequently contain calcifications that can be detected by plain radiography of the pelvis. Women who have gonadoblastomas often have ambiguous genitalia. The tumors are usually small and, in one-third of affected women, bilateral.

The malignant potential of immature teratomas correlates with the degree of immature or embryonic tissue present. The presence of choriocarcinoma can be determined histologically as well as by human chorionic gonadotropin (HCG) assays. The presence of choriocarcinoma in an immature teratoma worsens the prognosis.

Krukenberg's tumors are typically bilateral, solid masses of the ovary that nearly always represent metastases from another organ, usually the stomach. They contain large numbers of signet-ring adenocarcinoma cells within a cellular hyperplastic but nonneoplastic ovarian stroma.

497–500. The answers are: 497-B, 498-C, 499-D, 500-A. *(Novak, ed 8. pp 409–416, 485–490, 505–511, 532–530.)* Granulosa cell tumors show considerable microscopic variation. In most instances constituent cells resemble granulosa cells; and Call-Exner bodies, which are small liquefied cysts common in granulosa cells, may be observed in the better-differentiated forms of the tumor.

Arrhenoblastomas are malignant, masculinizing ovarian tumors. Testicular structures may be present (in the accompanying micrograph, testicularlike tubules can be observed). Reinke crystalloids also are often noted.

Benign cystic teratomas are the most common type of ovarian teratomas. The presence of sebaceous glandular elements are common; bone, cartilage, hair follicles, and skin also are frequently encountered.

Mucinous cystadenomas are characterized by the presence of the familiar, columnar, mucin-producing cell lining of the cyst cavity. No evidence of malignancy typically is found.

Bibliography

Aledjen S, Brown AK (eds): *Clinical Perinatology,* 2nd ed. St. Louis, CV Mosby, 1979.

American College of Obstetricians and Gynecologists: Suspect rape. *Am Coll Obstet Gynecol Tech Bull* 14:July, 1972.

American College of Obstetricians and Gynecologists: *Am Coll Obstet Gynecol Tech Bull* 61:3, 1981.

American Medical Association Committee on Human Sexuality: *Human Sexuality.* Chicago, American Medical Association, 1972.

Barden TP, Peter JB, Merkatz IR: Ritodrine hydrochloride: a betamimetic agent for use in preterm labor. I. Pharmacology, clinical history, administration, side effects, and safety. *Obstet Gynecol* 56:1–6, 1980.

Benirschke K: Twin placenta in perinatal mortality. *NY State J Med* 61:4499–4508, 1961.

Blaustein A (ed): *Pathology of the Female Genital Tract,* 2nd ed. New York, Springer-Verlag, 1982.

Burrow GN, Ferris TF (eds): *Medical Complications During Pregnancy,* 2nd ed. Philadelphia, WB Saunders, 1982.

Danforth DR: *Obstetrics & Gynecology,* 4th ed. Hagerstown, Harper & Row, 1983.

DiSaia PJ, Creasman WT: *Clinical Gynecologic 2nd ed. Oncology,* St. Louis, CV Mosby, 1984.

Gastel B, Haddow JE, Fletcher JC (eds): *Maternal Serum Alpha Fetoprotein: Issues in the Prenatal Screening and Diagnosis of Neural Tube Defects.* Washington, DC, US Government Printing Office, 1981.

Green TH Jr: *Gynecology: Essentials of Clinical Practice,* 3rd ed. Boston, Little Brown, 1977.

Jeanty P, Romero R: *Obstetrical Ultrasound.* New York, McGraw-Hill, 1984.

Jeffcoate N: *Principles of Gynecology,* 4th ed. Woburn, Mass., Butterworth, 1975.

Jones HW, Jones GS: *Novak's Textbook of Gynecology,* 10th ed. Baltimore, Williams & Wilkins, 1981.

Kase N, Weingold AB: *Principles of Clinical Gynecology.* New York, Wiley, 1983.

Lin CC, Evans MI: *Intrauterine Growth Retardation: Pathophysiology and Clinical Management.* New York, McGraw-Hill, 1984.

Masters WH, Johnson VE: *Human Sexual Inadequacy.* Boston, Little, Brown, 1970.

Masters WH, Johnson VE: *Human Sexual Response.* Boston, Little, Brown, 1966.

Mattingly RF: *Te Linde's Operative Gynecology,* 5th ed. New York, JB Lippincott, 1977.

Monif GR (ed): *Infectious Diseases in Obstetrics and Gynecology.* Hagerstown, Harper & Row, 1974.

Morrow CP, Townsend DE: *Synopsis of Gynecologic Oncology.* New York, Wiley, 1981.

Novak ER, Woodruff JD: *Novak's Gynecologic and Obstetric Pathology: With Clinical and Endocrine Relations,* 8th ed. Philadelphia, WB Saunders, 1979.

Parsons L, Sommers SC: *Gynecology,* 2nd ed. Philadelphia, WB Saunders, 1978.

Pritchard JA, MacDonald PC: *Williams Obstetrics,* 16th ed. New York, Appleton-Century-Crofts, 1980.

Queenan JT: *Modern Management of the RH Problem,* 2nd ed. Hagerstown, Harper & Row, 1977.

Romney SL, et al (eds): *Gynecology and Obstetrics: The Health Care of Women,* 2nd ed. New York, McGraw-Hill, 1981.

Ryan GM Jr (ed): *Ambulatory Care in Obstetrics and Gynecology.* New York, Grune & Stratton, 1980.

Sciarra JJ (ed): *Gynecology and Obstetrics,* 2nd ed. Hagerstown, Harper & Row. 1984.

Smith DW: *Recognizable Patterns of Human Malformation: Genetic, Embryologic, and Clinical Aspects.* Philadelphia, WB Saunders, 1982.

Speroff L, Glass RH, Kase NG: *Clinical Gynecologic Endocrinology and Infertility,* 3rd ed. Baltimore, Williams & Wilkins, 1983.

Therman E: *Human Chromosomes: Structure, Behavior, Effects.* New York, Springer-Verlag, 1980.

Thompson JS, Thompson MW: *Genetics in Medicine,* 3rd ed. Philadelphia, WB Saunders, 1980.

Vandenberg RI: Postpartum depression. *Clin Obstet Gynecol* 23:1105–1111, 1980.

Williams RH (ed): *Textbook of Endocrinology,* 6th ed Philadelphia, WB Saunders, 1982.

Wynn RM: *Obstetrics and Gynecology: The Clinical Core,* 3rd ed. Philadelphia, Lea & Febiger, 1983.

Yen SS, Jaffe RB (eds): *Reproductive Endocrinology: Physiology, Pathophysiology and Clinical Management.* Philadelphia, WB Saunders, 1978.